MANAGEMENT OF ACUTE TRAUMA

From the Continuing Education Course on the Management of Acute Trauma, The American Trauma Society, Atlanta, Georgia

MANAGEMENT OF ACUTE TRAUMA

Edited by

Herbert J. Proctor, M.D.

Professor of Surgery and Head, Trauma Section
University of North Carolina School of Medicine
Chapel Hill, North Carolina

Published by

Symposia Specialists Inc.
MEDICAL BOOKS

Distributed by

YEAR BOOK MEDICAL PUBLISHERS
CHICAGO • LONDON

A HOME STUDY TEXTBOOK PROGRAM

This book approved for
Category II Accreditation

The Seal that Guarantees You
Symposia Specialists Inc
The Best in Continuing Education

The American Trauma Society designates that this continuing medical education activity meets the criteria for **16 CREDIT HOURS IN CATEGORY II FOR THE PHYSICIAN'S RECOGNITION AWARD** of the American Medical Association *provided it is used and completed according to the instructions.*

To obtain the final examination, see colored insert at inside back cover.

Symposia Specialists, Inc.
1470 N.E. 129th Street
Miami, FL 33161

Distributed by
Year Book Medical Publishers
35 E. Wacker Drive
Chicago, IL 60601

Library of Congress Catalog Number 79-53674
International Standard Book Number 0-8151-6854-3

Printed in the United States of America

Contents

PANEL: EMT-PARAMEDIC TRAINING PROGRAMS

Preface

If there were a medical emergency right now, how many of you would know the appropriate emergency ambulance number to call? Probably about 95% would not know. As Emergency Medical Service advocates and practitioners, it is important that we practice what we preach.

In Emergency Medical Services (EMS) we tend to gravitate to those issues that either "yell" the loudest or have the most "sex" appeal. In other words, subjects such as advanced life support and EMT-Paramedics compel the most interest by not only the provider of EMS, but the consumer as well. Yes, it is nice to have the image or be part of the dramatic "life saver" role created by television and films. However, what is sometimes forgotten is that basic life support, as well as basic EMS systems concepts, is 90% of the action and will continue to be responsible for most lives saved in the pre-hospital phase of care.

Thus, the intent of this volume is for you to learn not only new ideas, skills and concepts, but also to be part of an extensive review of the basics. These basics will include airway management, fractures, patient stabilization and the role of the Emergency Medical Technician in EMS, as viewed from the standpoint of the 15 EMS components.

Though good patient care skills are essential for all of us, so too is the need to understand the system we work in and are a part of. Should you, as a good health care provider, know why you take a patient to a particular hospital? No, not just from the standpoint that the hospital is there, but from the concern that the hospital's care capability is most appropriate for the presenting injuries of your patient. Vertical categorization deals with this specific systems concept.

This volume has been developed to help you understand EMS a little better, as well as to review patient care skills. The American Trauma Society is well aware of the importance of

Emergency Medical Services and hopes that this volume will prove helpful.

Jeffrey S. Harris, REMT
Executive Director,
National Association of
Emergency Medical Technicians

Introduction

The idea of the American Trauma Society was first discussed at a meeting of the Committee on Shock of the National Research Council held in Washington, D.C., in 1964.

The magnitude of the trauma problem had been recognized, but no organized, concerted effort had been made to spearhead a fight against accidental injury. Fatalities due to injury had been steadily rising, until at that time trauma was the leading cause of death in persons from 1 to 37 years of age and the fourth leading cause of all deaths. Annually, accidental injuries were killing more than 100,000 persons, temporarily disabling over 10 million and permanently disabling over 400,000 Americans.

At the above meeting, I recommended that a two-pronged attack against trauma be launched: (1) the creation of a National Institute of Trauma within the framework of the National Institutes of Health and (2) the formation of an independent voluntary health organization to be known as the American Trauma Society. That was in 1964.

Working within the framework of the National Research Council, a Task Force consisting of Dr. Alan P. Thal, Dr. Sam F. Seeley, Dr. Joseph K. Owen and Dr. Howard developed a document entitled, "Accidental Death and Disability: The Neglected Disease of Modern Society." This was presented to the Committees on Trauma, Shock, and Anesthesia of the National Research Council and, with their endorsement, published by the National Academy of Science — National Research Council in 1966. Within this document was the recommendation that there be created an American Trauma Society as a voluntary health organization to parallel the role of The American Cancer Society and the American Heart Association in the field of accidental death and disability — an organization to involve the ambulance field, physicians, scientists, nurses, safety organizations, legislators, communication experts and, most of all, the public.

On May 11, 1967, at a meeting of the American Surgical Association at Colorado Springs, Colorado, Dr. Jonathan E. Rhoads convened an ad hoc group of surgeons to consider the concept of the American Trauma Society. With their support, he convened a special meeting in Philadelphia on July 8, 1967, when 32 distinguished Americans, predominantly from the surgical fields, decided to proceed with plans for organization. A certificate of incorporation of the American Trauma Society as a nonprofit corporation was formally filed in the State of Delaware June 27, 1968. The proposed charter included the following purposes:

"To inform the public of and to obtain its support for the corporation's activities in the field of trauma which shall be undertaken and carried on to:

(a) Assist and cooperate with medical, scientific, legal and nonprofit organizations interested in trauma and the prevention of injuries anywhere in the world and to encourage international cooperation in this field for the benefit of mankind.

(b) Encourage and foster research in the field of trauma and the education and training of persons in order to qualify them to engage in medical and scientific research in that field, the results of research to be made available to medical personnel engaged in the medical and surgical treatment of injuries.

(c) Encourage and foster, and voluntarily to assist financially and otherwise, the equipping, maintenance and operation of hospitals, clinics, laboratories and other facilities for the study and treatment of trauma.

(d) Collect, collate and make available statistical information relative to the incidence, mortality and treatment of personal injuries resulting from trauma.

(e) Encourage the creation of community programs to prevent injuries, improve the care of the injured and minimize the disability resulting therefrom.

(f) To cause to be established, as from time to time may be deemed desirable, associated or affiliated organizations to be designated "Divisions" and having substantially the same purposes and authorized by the corporation; and, by agreements with the Divisions, to assist in carrying out those purposes in defined geographical areas within the United States, its territories and dependencies; to renew, continue or terminate such agreements.

(g) Solicit and accept contributions of money and property, including but without limiting the generality of the foregoing, grants from Foundations and Federal or other governmental sources and to accept devises and bequests and all property received through trusts, endowments, deeds of gift, annuities, policies of insurance or otherwise, and to use and administer such property for the furtherance of these corporate purposes.

(h) Educate and train such persons as physicians, surgeons, hospital personnel, police and public health officers and personnel in techniques for the treatment and comfort of persons who have suffered trauma.

In the ten years since the Articles of Incorporation were filed in 1968, the Society has made a strong beginning. Today a new sense of confidence and momentum exists. Thirty-four State Divisions have been incorporated. Three thousand Founding Members have contributed to the financial initiation of the Society, a central office with a small but efficient staff has been developed in Chicago. A strong Board of Directors, consisting of outstanding physicians and community leaders, has accepted the responsibility for promoting the goals of the Society. With the Honorable Richard B. Ogilvie as Chairman of the Board of Directors and Miss Susan Weed as Executive Director of the Society, program-oriented Committees have been appointed, missions have been defined and programs are under way. This national symposium which we are initiating today represents part of the overall program organized by the Committee on Professional and Paraprofessional Training.

This year marks the end of the first decade of the Society, during which the foundation for growth has been developed. The coming decade should see evidence of tremendous momentum, spreading influence and improved care of the injured victim.

John M. Howard, M.D.
President, American Trauma Society

Public Relations in Emergency Care

Janet L. Schwettman, B.A.

Objectives

1. To differentiate between public relations, public information and public education.
2. To list pitfalls to be avoided in establishment of public relations programs.
3. To identify six mechanisms and four approaches applicable to good public relations programs.
4. To state reasons for increased patient interest in his medical problems.

Let us begin by differentiating between public relations, public information and public education — three rather lacklustre terms. *Public relations* refers to information transmitted to raise awareness, win support and promote goodwill. Broadly speaking, public relations really includes everything people *feel* about your organization or activity. *Public information* provides factual data to inform the public. *Public education* may provide information, training and technical skills, but its goal is modification of the attitudes, beliefs and behavior of the target group [1]. There is overlapping of each area, but this report will concentrate on public relations, presenting it in terms of modern day tugs and pulls.

In this age of consumerism, the medical world is placing new emphasis on the three areas just defined. This stems primarily from a reactionary stance, necessitated by public demand and the threat of litigation. If we consider why people are more concerned about their body, its problems and

Janet L. Schwettman, B.A., Community Relations Director, National Registry of Emergency Medical Technicians, Columbus, Ohio.

functions, it may aid us in developing a more creative public relations approach.

Public relations in the world of medicine was handed a staggering blow when the physician stopped making house calls, but it received a tremendous boost when the EMT began to respond to house, street, restaurant, or wherever calls, bringing basic and advanced life support to the side of the ill and injured.

The very act of *being* there is a powerful built-in public relations mechanism far beyond any campaign that Madison Avenue could ever create. At the scene of the incident, as the patient's first contact with medical personnel, the trained EMT makes an immediate, important impact. We should note that the message the EMT is capable of carrying goes beyond the treatment of the victim's medical problem and encompasses all facets of public relations. We have defined public relations as "information transmitted to raise awareness, win support and promote goodwill." While this is surely not the primary thrust of the EMT's vocation, the ripple effect exists. His actions in handling himself in a professional manner, as well as managing the patient, have become the *single most important facet of public relations in the prehospital emergency care setting . . .* for there is nothing more *public* than the locale of much of the EMT's action and nothing more potentially affirmative than the relationship established between the EMT and those he serves.

The consumer is well aware of the need for quality medical services and knows that this comes through sound, monitored education of health care personnel. Recognition of Nationally Registered EMTs across the country grows daily. Consumers gain confidence by knowing that a Nationally Registered EMT has met uniform, nationally acceptable standards, that continuing education requirements for reregistration must be met to maintain registered status and that a revocation for cause procedure has been established.

"Professional" is an *earned* label. It is perhaps sometimes too loosely applied to this newest of the allied health careers, the emergency medical technician. *American Heritage Dictionary* defines a professional as "one who has an assured level of competence in a particular field or occupation . . . ." Nationally Registered EMTs fit this definition, since they are measured at both the basic and advanced level in terms of training, experience and successful completion of both written and practical examinations, and they are held accountable for their actions.

Besides the on-scene public relations "message modality," the EMT has additional opportunities to impact, limited only by the amount of time he is willing and able to give. As you are aware, most ambulance service in this country is based in fire departments where personnel work 24/48 or 24/24 shifts or on a volunteer on-call basis. Therefore, in addition to being the nation's most visible health care provider functioning in the field, the EMT usually has another vocation and touches our lives not only when ambulance service is sought, but when the plumbing needs attention, the yards need landscaping, or any of the myriad services his other career provides. His "other career" contacts are excellent opportunities to move the EMS message as he interacts with his business clientele.

It is precisely because of this multiple role in society that the EMT can be a highly effective disseminator of EMS public relations. Interaction with the community occurs frequently in three ways other than ambulance service: as a business person, as a community oriented citizen and as a private individual. The whole personage of the EMT is a unique and valuable combination.

The EMT can be a refreshing speaker as well. He is a welcome relief at the monthly meetings of various organizations, for he has an exciting message to impart that holds the audience's attention. The EMT can also be importantly involved in those special EMS occasions, such as health fairs, Paramedic Days, EMS Week, etc. The list is endless for its focal point is the EMT himself. A tested tenet for establishing EMS systems is to "build on existing resources." Well, the EMT *exists* and is a tremendous resource upon which to build good public relations.

The types of interaction between hospital emergency departments and emergency medical technicians vary greatly, ranging from hospitals that simply receive the patient and the EMT immediately leaves to medical facilities which not only have EMTs assist in patient care in the Emergency Department, but also have regular inhospital follow-up contact between EMT, attending physician and patient. As stated in the text *Emergency Care and Transportation of the Sick and Injured*:

"There is no better way in which the EMT can learn to appreciate the extent to which his care influences full recovery or aids in reducing the degree of lasting disability than to observe the continuation of care by staff members in the emergency areas of a hospital." However it is handled or whoever is involved, each step in the movement of a patient in the hospital setting should be viewed as an opportunity to promulgate good relations. It is impressive and comforting to the patient to observe efficient teamwork. The smooth interaction of EMTs, nurses and physicians spells out true continuum of care, resulting in quality medical support, and is a psychological, emotional and intellectual plus for the victim of accident and illness. Verbal and nonverbal communications between EMTs, nurses and physicians are observed by the patient to a greater degree than generally acknowledged. Building the public's respect for the emergency health care team as a whole can be aided by awareness of this fact through the observance of common courtesies.

Each point of interaction between ED personnel and patient, family, or friends presents an opportunity for education, information and/or public relations. The chain of interpersonal, face-to-face communications in an emergency incident begins in the field — at the scene — as the EMT treats the patient and deals with family, neighbors, bystanders and often firemen and police. Upon arrival at the Emergency Department, patient contact may occur with admitting clerk, nurses, physician, ED support staff, family, friends, clergy, hospital ombudsman and, upon occasion, representatives from the press, television and radio.

Good communication by ED personnel with all who utilize the ED setting is not only considerate, but just plain smart business. The Robert Wood Johnson Foundation recently released its Final Report on the 44 sites the foundation funded from 1974 through 1977. The report included these words: "In the final analysis, EMS system continuance will depend on public acceptance and support. This presupposes a high quality of service; public awareness of the service and of how to use it; immediate and personal attention to all inquiries and complaints; complete openness of the operation to political, press, and public scrutiny; and a willingness to spend innumerable hours talking with rescue squads, county commissioners, civic clubs, hospital administrators, and physicians. Among the 44 projects, there appears to be a positive correlation between the time so spent and EMS system success."

Many hospitals have clergy in the ED for the benefit of the patient, family and EMTs. Because of their interest, some members of the clergy have taken EMT training and bring an added dimension to the role they play. Being part of the medical setting is also a beneficial learning experience for the clergy.

We are all aware of the tools which can be utilized in public relations and information programs — the media, printed material, word of mouth, billboards, bumper stickers, etc. But it is *people* who put it all together, and placing a live, unfettered, empathetic, experienced, creative mind in the PR coordination slot is top priority.

In conclusion, I'd like to leave you with four "rules" of the public relations road:

1. Apply imagination, avoid the "stapler mentality" that feeds in a standard idea, fastens it down and that ends the thinking process. In themselves, the terms "public education" and "information" lack sparkle, and "public relations" is a trite phrase, but the mechanisms can be bright and beautifully effective. For example, senior citizens in a condominium in northern Illinois held a paramedic gala, charged $5 a drink and raised $7,000 in one night for ambulance equipment while at the same time making the public aware of the advanced life support program's operational aspects. Personally, I learned so much that night from the most unappreciated segment of our society, the elderly. The senior citizens invited emergency physicians, nurses and EMTs who "public-related" themselves for hours as they conversed with elected officials and other members of the community.

There are so many organizations and individuals who would be delighted, honored, to be asked to be a part of any public relations program you develop. Once you initiate the project, you will be amazed at the enthusiasm generated and the original ideas that spring forth to accomplish the goals you seek.

2. Do not assume anyone knows anything about emergency medical services. Even the most meaningful and well-presented messages get fractured in the shuffle of our busy, noisy,

distracting world. Spell it out in a simplistic fashion and *continuously* program your efforts. The transient nature of today's world makes this mandatory. It is an unnecessary tragedy for a new resident to die or suffer needlessly when he moves into an area that has effective EMS of which he is unaware. Check to see if your message is getting across in a lasting manner. Polls are valuable and the results may surprise you, can guide you and in themselves are a good public relations mechanism. Random telephone polls utilizing volunteers as the work force, newspaper clip-and-send-in questionnaires, and homeroom polls in the schools are enlightening. Your methods need not be expensive to be effective.

3. Momentumize your timetable. Block out your goals, strategy and mechanisms, and see that milestones are established and met. Once lost, momentum is hard to retrieve.

4. Inject humor into your program. It is a common denominator for whatever we do in life. People relate to it, understand it and appreciate it. In the interaction of EMS personnel and the patient and his family, gentle humor can often be effective in reducing anxiety and impatience and can be catalytic in establishing the comfortable public relations we all seek.

Reference

1. EMS Public Information Guidebook. Philadelphia:NEMSIC, July 1978.

Self-Evaluation Quiz

1. Broadly speaking, public relations really includes:
   a) Everything people feel about your organization or activity
   b) Factual data to inform the public
   c) Information and technical skills
   d) None of the above
2. The single, most important facet of public relations in the prehospital emergency care setting is:
   a) A 911 system
   b) A quick response time by the EMT
   c) The EMT's action in handling himself and the patient in a professional manner
   d) Good relationship with newspaper reporters

3. Ambulance personnel who are Nationally Registered:
    a) Are all members of fire departments
    b) Must be 21 years of age
    c) Have met uniform, nationally acceptable standards and must meet continuing education requirements
4. Interaction between EMT and hospital Emergency Department personnel:
    a) Should be held to a minimum
    b) Should give the EMT an opportunity to observe the continuation of care by staff members in the emergency areas of the hospital
    c) Is basically unimportant if a good training program is operational
    d) Is not observed by the patient
5. Which of the following is the most important when initially putting together a public relations program?
    a) Bumper stickers
    b) Word of mouth
    c) Billboards
    d) Creative PR director

Answers on page 289.

Legal Aspects of Pre-Hospital Care

Arthur M. Kaplan

Objectives

1. To understand the specific role of the EMT and why sometimes this role should be reduced.
2. To realize that the EMT is not a physician and requires continuous supervision to prevent legal and medical difficulties.
3. To define emergency situations and what is meant by implied consent.

I have been privileged to be a part of the emergency medical system for almost 20 years. I have seen changes that are almost unbelievable. Thousands of lives have been preserved and injuries minimized by the EMT by adequate emergency care, not only in Atlanta, but all over Georgia and in many other states. It is amazing that in a few short years the EMT profession could be conceived and then developed so rapidly and extensively. It is gratifying because it shows what people can and will do when called upon to respond. The EMT system is one of the greatest developments that has emerged in the emergency care field. How many of these people would not have survived were it not for the care rendered by EMTs. Someone asked me recently if I was opposed to advanced life support. I am all for advanced life support. I think it is a necessary and very integral part of the totality of emergency care if it is properly implemented by adequately trained personnel who possess sufficient maturity, knowledge, training and background to assume this awesome responsibility.

Today, society and the medical profession are in a crisis unparalleled and unheralded to any known in the history of the

---

Arthur M. Kaplan, Judge, Municipal Court of Atlanta; EMT Instructor, Atlanta, Ga.

medical profession. Physicians and those in other professions are being sued frivolously. What would have happened 20 to 25 years ago if this had occurred? Malpractice suits were virtually unheard of. You could not get one physician to testify against another. There was a physician to physician loyalty. Today we receive brochures almost daily which say in effect: "Submit your medical claim to us for possible litigation and let us review the files and prepare your case." We get similar literature from all over the country. A recent issue of the *Emergency Medical Technician Legal Bulletin* tells of law actions, law suits, that are developing. I have a few cases stemming primarily from California, which I shall return to momentarily.

The EMT and the emergency medical care field are really embryonic when you consider the many years of medical care, training and research that have preceded their birth. In reality, the advanced emergency care in this country is almost in a state of ventricular fibrillation.

Physicians give orders to people they consider to be competent, but they know not who these people are. All they know is a voice over the telephone or radio calling for medical care, not basic care, but medical care — starting of intravenous fluids, defibrillation, cardiac drugs, thoracotomy tubes in the chest, esophageal airways, endotracheal tubes. They are asking a physician in an emergency room for permission to do these procedures. To whom is the physician responding?

The patient must be assessed in most instances not by the physician but by the EMT who transmits his findings to the physician. The physician must then respond, based upon this series of symptoms or assessments by the EMT. To be an EMT in Georgia and in most states, one must be 18 years of age. There is no requirement for a college background, just the sole age requirement. One then takes a 125- or 150-hour course in emergency care, which is a good course, a good start. Then one is an EMT, authorized to administer basic first aid on an ambulance, dependent upon passing a certain test and meeting certain qualifications.

EMT-Paramedics have had a certain degree of definitive and practical experience. They have worked in the emergency room, intubated a few patients, started one or possibly two dozen or maybe even 100 intravenous fluids. He is given a minimal amount of training with reference to drugs, their effects, uses, indications and, to some extent, contraindications. Then he goes out into the field and radios his message to a physician: "Request to start protocol number one. I have a trauma patient involved in an automobile wreck, with a fractured femur, blood pressure is such and such, pulse is such and such, respiration is such and such." Then it is up to the physician to accept or reject this EMT's evaluation.

In other words, instead of the paramedic being subordinate to the physician, the physician is subordinate to the paramedic. It is almost the reverse of what it was actually intended to be. If the physician grants the procedure, then he is primarily responsible, based upon that paramedic's request and assessment of that patient. Has he drawn blood gases? Does he know the patient's history or his problems? Is he able to take a history and get some general idea from looking at this patient of some other underlying problems? No, the paramedic would have no idea. The physician has had four years of undergraduate college, four years of medical school and a minimum of four years internship and residency. So we are talking about 12 years versus 12 weeks. If the physician elects to give the medication desired and then something goes wrong, the physician has a problem. He is primarily the one that the patient, through his attorney, will hold responsible.

Now let us reverse the situation. This is something that is beginning to surface now, but there is a forerunner case in California. Let us suppose the physician says, "No, simply transport the patient to the hospital." There is something about the paramedic's assessment of this patient that makes the physician unsure of the proper or specific treatment for this patient. He has not seen that patient; perhaps he does not want to abide by the paramedic's assessment. So the physician replies to the paramedic, "Request denied." Then a problem develops. The paramedic says, "If the physician had let me do that, the patient would not have died." A postmortem autopsy is conducted. There are certain things that could have been done, perhaps definitively, which might have preserved the life of that patient, might, I say, might have, could have. Remember this word *could* because I shall refer to this shortly.

Now the physician is faced with another problem. He failed to respond to the paramedic's request. Does the physician have an inherent right to do this?

Registered Nurses have spent three or four years in nursing school, many hours of clinical care and patient observation. They do not have the authority that is being delegated to the paramedic. Nor does the physician's assistant have the authority delegated to the EMT. How will we overcome this dilemma? What are the implications?

Another problem that we are experiencing is friction and criticism of one another. The EMT does not like what the nurse did in the clinic. The nurse is dissatisfied with the way the EMT splinted a leg. The physician is a little bit harsh that it took so long to get the patient to the hospital. There is now revolving dissension and friction. We cannot tolerate that. It must be overcome by professionalism. Nevertheless, it exists. The physician envies the nurse, the nurse envies the EMT. Some people dislike a particular ambulance service. This presents, again, a degree of friction. In other words, you are not able to sit down calmly and collectively and discuss rationally the problems with the other party. They are not willing to give you the opportunity to face them and ask questions, such as, "Why did you do this?" On the contrary, they must talk behind your back. Finally, when they finish their conversation, the facts are altered so greatly you would not even believe it is the same incident any longer that you were involved with.

Unfortunately, we are forgetting the basics too often. We are jumping into the advanced too rapidly. We fail to maintain the airway manually. We fail to clear the mouth and remove the obstructed object from the mouth. No, we must immediately insert the endotracheal tube or the esophageal airway into the patient because that is the way physicians do it on television programs. Let me be the first to admit that the TV program "Emergency!" was the greatest assistance we have had because it served to educate the public. It showed just what can be done, but now we have another problem. Almost every time they come out of the unit, the defibrillator or EKG is in one hand and intravenous fluids in the other. If they do cardiopulmonary resuscitation, that is fine. I saw some of them doing it recently and they were doing compressions beautifully. They had only one small problem: they forgot to breathe the patient.

Let us consider endotracheal intubation. There was a case recently in California against the paramedics because they failed to recognize an obstruction and forced the obstruction deeper into the throat by the insertion of an endotracheal tube. You learn to intubate in a sophisticated environment: in the emergency room or in the operating room. You are now out at the scene. A person is having respiratory difficulty. You are able to bag the victim and get an airway going. It may not be the best airway in the world but you have a partial airway established and are getting an exchange of air. But we are determined to put in an endotracheal tube. By radio you tell the physician: "Labored breathing. Request permission to insert an endotracheal tube." The physician replies, "Permission granted." Then severe damage or trauma is done to that trachea. Perhaps it is ruptured. Had the physician bothered to ascertain (1) how close you were to the hospital — two, three, five or ten minutes away, (2) the accessibility of that patient or (3) if you had a table on which to place the patient to get him off of the ground, if he happened to be on the ground, so that you would have good access to the patient's trachea? In other words, was the position and area in which you were working on that patient conducive to successful endotracheal intubation? Did the physician ask these questions? I think not, and by virtue of that, trauma results.

I can truthfully say that I do not know who would be liable in that instance, but I can promise you somebody in the near future will find out because it is not feasible for an EMT to get down on the ground next to that victim and try to insert an endotracheal tube in the trachea in darkness. It is seldom successful. Even in the best environment and under controlled conditions the physician and the respiratory therapist have an awesome task to get that endotracheal tube inserted, especially if there is a spasm. Therefore, somebody had better take a second look at what you are doing.

What would the effects of a legal action be? I do not know. Some states have insurance requirements for EMTs. Most states, however, do not. What effect is it going to have on the physician? Is the physician's insurance going to cover him for delegating authority for the EMT to act? I do not know. The insurance covers the physician and his acts, but does his insurance cover him for yours? Perhaps you are someone he has never seen before, whose qualifications he has not determined. To him, you are simply and only a voice.

I read recently that the theory of my job is to make the best medical decision for the patient, not a legal decision for myself. If you do not take the legal aspect into consideration, there is not going to be an EMS system because the law will stop it. If you do not consider your acts, as to their propriety or impropriety, you had better start doing so now.

Are all EMTs equally competent? They are not. We have all different types of EMTs. We have some who are first rate in every community, and we have some who are decidedly inferior, who just barely got through their training. What are your problems with the EMT who is not nearly qualified if you happen to be working together with him in the back of an ambulance? Where do you stand in relation to his actions if what you do is correct and what he does is incorrect?

The topic "The Medical Intervenor" appeared in a recent issue of the *Emergency Medical Technician Legal Bulletin.* It alludes primarily to the person on the street who has assumed the emergency care of a victim. He is the intervenor. When you get to the scene and take over and the intervenor commits some detrimental act, if a suit is brought, it will be against both of you. It probably will not be brought against only one. It will be brought against everybody the plaintiff's lawyer can join in. They are known in law as joint tortfeasors.

Another subject is implied consent. Do we really understand what implied consent means? For all practical purposes, it is a consent to surgical or medical treatment or procedures suggested, recommended, prescribed or directed by a duly licensed physician and will be implied where an emergency exists. For the purposes of determining an emergency, it is a situation where (a) competent medical judgment, proposed surgical or medical treatment or procedure are reasonably necessary and (b) a person authorized to consent is not readily available and any delays in treatment could reasonably be expected to jeopardize the life or health of the person affected, or could reasonably result in disfigurement or impair faculties.

Let's look at the other side of the coin. Where does it end for the physician? Where does it end for the EMT? Does it authorize one to invade that victim's body with a thoracotomy tube? Does it delegate authority by some strange fashion of the law that says that the physician can authorize the EMT after certain weeks of training and certification to insert an endotracheal tube into the victim's trachea? Regardless of the particular Code Section where you might be granted this authority, there is considerable doubt in my mind, at this point, whether our legislators can constitutionally enact such legislation. This must be determined in the future by our judiciary.

Are we going too fast and too far in our embryonic stage? Should we reassess what we are doing and build and grow a little bit at a time? What kind of medical controls do we have? Do we have standing orders? Standing orders in Georgia are illegal. There is a great difference between a standing order and a medical protocol. A standing order means you are authorized to do what you think is appropriate, without first consulting with a physician. A medical protocol means you must get the order from the physician first to institute the protocol. This is a predetermined set of medical procedures, but you must still first obtain the order from that physician.

I have great respect for the EMT, for what he is doing and what he is trying to do. But there are some EMTs who get a dual certification when they obtain their EMT license. In the minds of some, they have been certified as an EMT and as a "junior" physician coincidental thereto. They are not "junior" physicians. The only way in which an EMT can be a physician is to graduate from a certified four-year medical school and complete medical training as a physician.

I have seen EMTs with hemostats attached to their coats, which resemble a series of railroad tracks. What are they going to do with all those hemostats? The EMT replies, "Well, I may have a bad hemorrhage." In what text has there ever been any mention of controlling a hemorrhage with a hemostat? It is not in there. This EMT may have had specific training from a very fine surgeon who perhaps told him all of the dangers of the hemostats: what to look for, what not to clamp, what should be clamped, to stay away from the nerves and not to clamp two or three vessels at one time simply in order to get to one and so forth. However, the EMT still has no authority to have them. There is no set standard procedure in our texts for this. It is an ego trip in most instances that the EMT is carrying around these hemostats.

I saw one EMT carrying a portable set of disposable scalpels — there must have been six scalpels sticking out of his pocket.

Whatever he was going to do would exceed the bounds of an EMT's authority with those instruments. For what intent and purposes did he have these instruments and what type of justification therefor?

I am not being disparaging of the EMT. If your partner exhibits this type of behavior, get rid of him. Do not get caught in the flypaper of negligence.

Another problem is the intermingling of orders. For example, a paramedic calls in on his radio to the physician in the hospital for a protocol on a patient. The physician authorizes him to implement the physician's orders. Does that mean that the physician also says that another EMT can do the same procedure as the first EMT? No, it does not. The order is applicable only to that individual to whom he granted that order because, ostensibly, that person to whom he granted that order has the legal authority to implement that physician's orders. It mentions nothing about someone else. In fact, anyone other than the EMT to whom the order was dispatched may be in violation of the criminal statutes of the state. He may be in violation of the medical practice act. He may be in violation of the dangerous drug act, being in possession of or administering a prescribed medication without the authority of a physician. The physician did not give him the order, or he may be guilty of a simple battery because what he did was illegal and without authority.

California enacted the first set of laws in the United States governing the EMS. These were the forerunners for emergency and other means of emergency care. I am grateful to California for enacting these, but they are getting a little bit concerned about lawsuits. Until today, I know of very few lawsuits that have been brought and plaintiff judgment rendered in a case pertaining to emergency care. Ironically, a case was brought in and decided in Georgia, where one of the defendants invoked the Good Samaritan act. This was a case in which a contractor's employee fell off a house. The owner and the contractor took him to his home and not to a hospital. The man sued the contractor and the owner, alleging that they should have taken him to a hospital and they should not have moved him. The owner invoked the Good Samaritan act, stating that her actions were in good faith and without compensation. The court in a summary judgment dismissed the case against the owner. The court of appeals upheld it. That is the only case of which I am aware, but there are many cases with reference to physicians.

Let us consider the enema. In this case, a female patient went to a physician some months or even years previous to this incident. They operated and removed a part of her colon. A cancer was diagnosed and the surgeon inserted a colostomy. The physician followed the progression of the growth until such time as he deemed it appropriate that a barium enema had to be administered. Until this time, they had administered the barium orally and followed her that way. The patient went to the physician's office. The x-ray technician, the radiologist and one other person inserted the tube into the colostomy. "Certainly, it is going to be painful," they told her when she began to complain of the discomfort. Despite her screams, they persisted. It was finally taken out. Several weeks later, the sheriff came to the physician's office. The lady through her attorney sued the physician, the technician, the radiologist and the other person for battery because they caused her to have serious, severe pain against her wishes. It took three weeks to try that case. The Court dismissed the charge against the physician's subordinates, but the physician had to stand trial. The jury was out for 30 minutes and then brought in a verdict for the defendant. This lady appealed the case and the Court of Appeals upheld the trial Court's judgment for the defendant.

California recently enacted a law in 1978 which says: "Emergency medical services and emergency medical care means those medical services required for the immediate diagnosis and treatment of medical conditions which if not immediately diagnosed and treated could lead to serious physical or mental disability or death." Notice that it does not say *would lead* but *could lead*. I do not know the lawyer who prepared this document or prepared this law, but I rather suspect he had some friends in the insurance industry because it is almost unconscionable. Further, in order to protect the interests of certain categories of people, primarily the paramedics, they enacted the following law: "He who renders emergency medical services at the scene of an emergency shall only be liable in civil damages for acts or omissions performed in a grossly negligent manner or not performed in good faith."

In most states, including Georgia, *slight diligence or gross negligence* is defined as follows: "Slight diligence or gross negligence. In general, slight diligence is that degree of care which every man of common sense howsoever inattentive he may be exercises under the same or similar circumstances, applies the preservation of property. Slight diligence means that care which every man of common sense howsoever inattentive he may be takes of his own property. The absence of such care is termed gross negligence."

It is hard to believe that legislators of California will let anyone, including the paramedic, come up to the scene of an accident and do just about anything short of being grossly negligent.

They attempted to vitiate the rights, abrogate the rights, the legal rights of victims. You cannot legislate away negligence. You cannot contract away negligence.

Yes, by virtue of this type of reasoning, I am opposed to advanced life support and you had better be also, because if you are not and we try to get acts like this passed, we are going to lose the EMS in this community and country unless the present advanced life support is reassessed and implemented under proper medical controls, and I do not mean medical controls of small communities, but national medical controls, and unless we get the professional people together and say: "This is what we will do and this is all that we will do and that is all you are authorized to do."

As long as you rely on the basics and perform them properly, you should have no legal problems. If there are not sufficient guidelines and medical control set down for the implementation of advanced care, demands are going to be made of you and you will be totally dominated and compelled into involuntary, ineffective, unsupported standards. You will be compelled, especially physicians, to do things against your better judgment which could conceivably place you in a very dangerous legal position. Unfortunately, your subordinates will also feel the implications thereof.

When you are on duty, working with your ambulance service, you are authorized to carry certain medications and drugs. What about when you are off duty? Do you have the authority to carry those medications and drugs with you in your privately owned automobile? No, you do not. They must be deposited at the hospital or other designated area in a properly prepared locker under safe supervision under the hospital's or other duly authorized authority.

How many have a federal license to possess and dispense medications and narcotics? Where do the drugs come from? What do you have in your ambulance? Who put them there? Under whose authority? If it happens that you have medications and narcotics in your possession in your privately owned automobile, you may very well be held guilty of a felony for illegal possession and control of narcotics.

Another problem is the time delay in administering the advanced care. In California, a man brought an action against the ambulance personnel for taking too much time to get his wife, who had a ruptured spleen, to the hospital. The men who arrived at the scene took a very long time deciding what to do for the victim. If she had been taken to the hospital, perhaps she could have been saved, but she died.

As for verbal orders, if a physician issues instructions to you, insist he write them down or give them over a tape-recorded communications system. If your system is neither written nor taped, you are going to have a problem because if something should develop and you do not have a permanent record of the order, either written or taped, then the physician can say, "I did not tell him to do that. I told him to do this!" The other man says, "Yes, I heard you, and you did not say that but you said this." Then it is a matter of evidence as to who said what to whom and when it was said. It is going to have to go before a jury. The nurse has no authority to convey the orders of the physician. I do not care what your hospital regulations say, I do not care what your hospital administrator says. If you call in for orders, the law says that it must be under the order of a physician. It does not say anything about the transmission of the order by the physician's nurse. If the legislators wanted that in there, they would have inserted it.

Self-Evaluation Quiz

1. The EMT should have a *specific* role in the care of emergency victims. According to the author this is to:

a) Act as a physician in urgent situations
b) Be able to make a diagnosis of common medical problems
c) Be well trained to maintain airways and to provide accurate descriptive data to the listening physician
d) Understand telemetry, drug administration and disease processes so as to act intelligently in emergency situations

2. A standing order means authorization to do what is appropriate without first consulting with a physician.
a) True
b) False

3. The author believes that the physician has been rendered subordinate to the EMT and is at risk of lawsuits.
a) True
b) False

Answers on page 289.

Panel: Career Future for the EMT

A. E. Hertzler Knox, M.D.
Michael Lummis
Chris Gentile

Introduction

A. E. Hertzler Knox, M.D.

The present field of emergency medical services is experiencing problems in the turnover rate of personnel. It has been estimated, for example, that the average working span for a paramedic in the Los Angeles system is approximately five years. Are these individuals leaving the work force because of the stress of their chosen career, low pay, because they were educated to expect more than the job has to offer, or because of the lack of the possibility of career advancement? The next two papers are designed to be complementary and are by two experts in the field of emergency medical services education and training. Michael Lummis will present the present educational and career ability aspects for emergency medical technicians and will address the questions as to whether the present educational system adequately prepares an individual for a career as an emergency medical technician and should individuals in emergency medical supervisory positions be drawn from the pool of emergency medical technicians thus created. To give added depth to Mr. Lummis's presentation Chris Gentile will suggest a modification of the present educational system for emergency medical technicians in order to provide a better opportunity for career advancement into multiple areas of emergency medical service and will suggest that this will possibly remedy the five-year "burnout" syndrome that many emergency medical systems are experiencing.

A. E. Hertzler Knox, M.D., Medical Director, Office of Emergency Medical Services, State Department of Health, Hartford, Conn.

Career Future for the EMT: Are Educational Techniques Responsible for "Burnout"?

Michael Lummis

Objectives

To understand the concepts, training and education and career-building aspects of emergency medical technician (EMT) field and supervisory positions among the other allied medical areas of service.

I shall begin my remarks by stating that I believe that EMT-A and EMT-P, as they exist today, do not offer significant potential for a traditional long-term career. While there are obvious exceptions, this premise applies to the vast majority of the EMT-A and EMT-P personnel who are currently active in the Emergency Care System in America. This lack of career opportunity is not limited to the field level personnel in EMS, but rather is typical of the entire system. In other words, I do not believe that *any* realistic opportunities exist for large numbers of persons to build traditional careers in *any* jobs in EMS. An example of this premise is found in the program of this symposium, where the presenters for this session are Chris Gentile and myself. We have been involved in EMS for some time. If we could retreat in time to January 16, 1973, when Richard M. Nixon announced his EMS initiative, and follow the career paths of these two individuals, we would find that multiple distinct positions have been held by this small group in just five years. It is also interesting that one of us has changed

---

Michael Lummis, Instructor, Emergency Medical Training, University of Kansas Medical Center, Kansas City.

positions in the past month. Further evidence of the instability of EMS positions is found when one investigates the top EMS training positions in each state. The National Council of Emergency Medical Training Directors has identified 40 such positions in America. Between February 15, 1978, and October 15, 1978, there were personnel changes in 14 of the 40 positions, for a net turnover of 35%. With this track record, one might speculate that another top EMS administrative position is changing hands, even as we meet here in Atlanta.

Because I do not believe that this job instability is limited to administrative positions, I would like to cite figures from my home state of Kansas, relating to the numbers of active field personnel. The primary efforts to train EMT-A personnel in Kansas started on May 9, 1974. Since that time, more than 5,400 EMT-A personnel have been trained in Kansas. Out of this group, approximately 4,200 are currently certified, representing a turnover of more than 20%.

It is appropriate to give a great deal of consideration to the questions that logically follow such statistics. Why do we find such a high rate of turnover in EMS? Why is EMS lacking in employment stability? Finally, can anything be done to combat these problems?

I believe that a primary source of these problems can be found in the educational/training component of EMS, which is a unique component, dissimilar to the educational/training components of any other allied health vocation. This uniqueness is worth taking a second look in order to understand its nature. Most traditional allied health vocations are developed through the traditional, or pedagogic educational system. Most people who enter an allied health field participate in pedagogic educational pursuits from the age of 6 until they complete their education/training and enter their chosen allied health vocation. Pedagogy is a term that liberally translated simply means "education by banking." This approach is the traditional passage of knowledge from one generation to the next. The pedagogic educator simply states: "I have the knowledge, and I will give it to you." Pedagogy is the foundation of our educational system.

The growth of EMS occurred too rapidly for meaningful education/training within the framework of a pedagogic system.

Most of those who have entered EMS in the past five years are adults. In fact, one could speculate that the vast majority of those who have come into the field in the past five years are adults. Since the majority are adults, it seems logical to assume that the majority have been away from the traditional educational/training system for a significant period of time and cannot be considered as pedagogic learners.

The science of adult education, or Andragogy, is a relatively new development in education, but nevertheless, strong evidence exists to indicate that adults require a different educational/training approach than do children. This is even more pronounced when the adult has been away from the pedagogic educational/training system for a significant period of time.

Those who promote the andragogic viewpoint have cited three primary motivating factors that bring the adult into a learning situation. The first, and perhaps the most common factor that brings an adult into a learning situation is that the learning is required. I believe we can all recognize that many EMT-A and EMT-P personnel have been trained because the training was required for continuing employment.

A second motivating factor that brings the adult into a learning situation is the desire to socialize. I am certain that trainers will agree that many people show up in an EMT-A class because their friends and neighbors are there and an opportunity to interact socially is offered. This is particularly true in the voluntary setting, and is not necessarily limited to EMS. A similar situation exists in volunteer fire services and law enforcement agencies.

A third motivating factor that has been identified is the commitment of the life-long learner, who will repeatedly place himself in a learning situation, based on a desire to acquire knowledge.

Each of these factors presents unique problems that must be dealt with effectively if an adult is to be placed in a learning situation that becomes a long-term commitment. The failure of our system to recognize significant differences between educating children and training adults has contributed significantly to the high rate of turnover within the field. The EMT-A or EMT-P must be committed to life-long learning, and we have failed to develop adequate mechanisms to insure that those who enter the field of EMS are suitable candidates for such a commitment. Because this approach is in error from the beginning, there is no margin for individual consideration, and those who are not motivated internally are soon lost, at great cost to our system.

I believe that this failure to recognize new candidates for EMS positions, particularly field positions, as adults, is particularly important, but I also believe that another basic mistake has been made in our educational/training approach. I hope that this belief, as well as the remarks that I have already made, will lead to informed debate in order that we can make some degree of progress.

EMS is, and has been, a rapidly growing and changing phenomenon. In essence, I believe that our educational/training component has been created as a dilution of medical education. Usually, our approach to the student EMT-A or EMT-P has been to start with the basic sciences and progress through anatomy and physiology to specific body systems and specific injuries and/or disorders. This approach assumes that an EMT-A or EMT-P must understand the mechanism of oxygen exchange at the cellular level in order to adequately deal with a nonbreathing patient. I would submit that it is ridiculous to require the EMT-A or EMT-P to understand the oxygenation status of blood in systemic or pulmonary circulation, simply because he will be required to perform basic and/or advanced life support. I would also challenge anyone to justify the necessity for an EMT to understand the microcellular aspects of hypovolemic shock as a prerequisite to dealing with a traumatized patient. Nevertheless, a visit to any EMT-A or EMT-P training center will confirm that we are spending huge amounts of time on such mundane and inappropriate topics.

In order to overcome these problems, I would propose a utilization of existing patient assessment and patient care algorithms, which have now been available for several years. The use of such algorithms can develop an EMT-A or EMT-P who deals with patient assessment in an orderly, logical sequence that is patient oriented, rather than focused on only a part or single system of the patient. Once a technician is adequately trained in the use of the algorithms, and programs are established to implement a patient-centered approach, field care of the sick and injured might be maintained at highly competent levels through the maintenance of psychomotor skills.

A humanist might argue that such an approach is technical, degrading, and would eventually create a higher turnover rate than we are already experiencing. Conversely, I would assert that anyone who carefully examines the day-to-day field care that is offered at the EMT-A and EMT-P level will find that most patient care follows the algorithmic pattern, despite the dichotomous nature of current training. In other words, we are training people to think, but in effect, they are required to act. Jobs become a series of technical skills, repeated in a variety of situations, as dictated by patient assessment. Since we have educated/trained the field personnel to think and to "diagnose," is it any wonder that we are faced with high turnover and technician "burnout"?

We are now faced with the fact that the idea of a career ladder, or career tract, has been developed as a remedy for turnover and "burnout." We are, in effect, saying: "Let's give these people some administrative expertise, and they will get motivated." Unfortunately, there are some serious questions in regard to training EMS Administrators. First, where are the administrative jobs for these people? What is the present status of career ladders that will allow for upward mobility? There are a few obvious answers, particularly in those Emergency Services that exist as a part of fire services. One might project that the security, benefits and retirement plans offered by most fire services will attract a number of EMT-A and EMT-P personnel to long-term employment. One might also speculate that a large number of dedicated volunteer EMT-A personnel, particularly in rural areas, will maintain long-term certification. On the whole, however, I must conclude that there are not significant numbers of traditional careers in EMS that are open under our present system.

As an alternative to current thinking, I would like to propose an alternate methodology for those interested in careers in EMS. I will first direct my attention to the arena of administration and management and then turn to the field of education/training.

Current thinking indicates that a career in EMS should progress from the EMT-A level to the EMT-P level, and then into supervision, midmanagement and, finally, management/administration. As a part of this "career ladder," the EMT-A component is seen as a component of the EMT-P program. I believe that this is totally unrealistic. I would agree that EMT-A training is a prerequisite for an EMT-P program, but under our current system of training, there is no orderly progression from the basic sciences of the EMT-A to the extensive anatomy and physiology that is currently required of the EMT-P. If our system was based on the algorithmic approach, starting with patient assessment and progressing to specific patient care modalities, a progression from EMT-A to EMT-P would be possible. An EMT-P would simply proceed further through the protocols prescribed through the algorithm. There would be no differences in the basic algorithm.

Under the current system, a great many people seem to hold the opinion that an effective supervisor, midmanager or administrator must possess an EMT-P certification. I believe that this position is equally untenable. There is no question that EMT-P crews require EMT-P supervisors, but the amount of training necessary for this function has nothing to do with the basic certification. If we are to build a system based on sound administration, then the emphasis must be on developing administrative skills, and the EMT-P certification does not endow any individual with *any* basic administrative skills. In other words, if the system is to achieve maturity, we must recognize the need for skilled administrators, who will be judged on their administrative skills, and not on their degree of certification at the field level.

The example of the private practice of medicine illustrates the last point. During the past decade, the most pronounced change in medical practice has been the growth of large specialty and multispecialty clinics. These clinics are administered by trained administrators, whose knowledge of medicine is rudimentary. In other words, physicians are not providing administrative direction for their own practices, but rather rely on a trained administrator with some understanding of health care services. Nationally, there are two professional organizations for clinic managers, the American Association of Medical Clinics and the Medical Group Management Association, as well as a certification body, the American College of Clinic Managers. I am therefore proposing that EMS Administrators need to be knowledgeable about the field, but not necessarily certified at an advanced level.

Many of our mid to upper level managers and administrators have come into the system from the "Grandfather" network, through their prior association with ambulance services and other previous providers of emergency services. Many of these people are going to be in the system for several years to come. One particular need that we must address in a meaningful manner is the development of educational programs for these incumbents. A number of organizations, including the National Association of Emergency Medical Technicians, and several universities are moving in this direction, so perhaps progress is being made.

I believe that a viable alternative to baccalaureate EMS administration programs may also be presented by the growth and development of degree programs in Allied Health. Emergency Medical Services are certainly a part of the overall Allied Health occupations, and a Bachelor of Science degree is the logical entry point for someone wishing to pursue administration. A degree of this type also provides a logical "career ladder" into advanced degree programs, such as the Masters in Public Administration, the Masters in Community Health or the Masters in Health Administration.

To summarize my remarks concerning an alternate approach to EMS Administration, I would recommend that we develop tracts for the continuing education of incumbent EMS administrators and that we develop tracts within Bachelors of Science programs, in Allied Health, as a future entry level administrative program in EMS.

My thoughts concerning education are similar. We must develop an educational tract within EMS that provides a career ladder within the overall educational system. While I believe that a great deal of emphasis must be devoted to andragogic skills and techniques, we must also be prepared to change, if new entry into the field level of EMS becomes a part of the pedagogic system. We need to develop tracts within existing Educational degree programs that provide meaningful skills for EMS trainers and educators, and we must provide the opportunity for these persons to fit into the existing Masters and Ph.D. programs in Education.

In conclusion, I believe that we do not currently have a meaningful career ladder within EMS. We must also recognize that we are currently experiencing a critical level of "burnout," or turnover. I would place a great deal of the blame for this phenomenon on the educational/training methodology that is utilized by the system. I have suggested an alternate approach, utilizing the algorithmic approach, but I believe it is particularly critical that we examine all possible alternatives. In the meantime, we must stop telling people that they are entering a traditional career field and provide them with realistic information concerning long-term opportunities. We must reexamine our thinking in regard to EMS Administration and concentrate on providing skills for incumbent administrators. We must plan for the future through the development of meaningful, comprehensive administrative tracts that place emphasis on administration, rather than technical skills.

Self-Evaluation Quiz

1. According to the author, EMS offers:
   a) Long-term careers
   b) Nothing at all today
   c) Limited advancement
   d) An opportunity to transfer to medical school
2. EMS field personnel:
   a) Are trained physicians or equivalent
   b) Are trained nurses or equivalent
   c) Are trained firemen-rescue personnel types
   d) Cannot build long-term careers
3. EMS positions are:
   a) Relatively stable if you are easily satisfied
   b) Generally unstable
   c) Stable under all conditions if you have an M.D. degree
   d) Eagerly sought after by nurses who fail licensing exams
4. The National Council of Emergency Medical Training has identified _____ top training positions:
   a) 40 per state
   b) 5 in the United States
   c) 40 in the United States
5. What was the turnover (attrition rate) of the personnel in question 4?

a) None
b) 8%
c) 20%
d) 35%

6. EMT job stability is limited to administrative positions.
   a) True
   b) False

Answers on page 289.

Career Future for the EMT: The Case for the Associate Degree

Chris Gentile

Objectives

To consider the semantics, conceptualization and training aspects of emergency medical technician careers in a changing context of medical care.

In terms of the development of career capability in emergency medical services, I think we must first look at where it all started. At about the turn of the decade, we started training emergency medical technicians (EMTs). Of course, nobody knew what they were, who they were, what they could do or where they were going. At that time, there were probably no more than a handful of paramedic programs and the criteria of those themselves were somewhat diversified in their definitions. The problems that immediately faced the new profession: What was an EMT? What is an EMT? How did the EMT relate to some of the more common terms of the time, such as an ambulance attendant, a medical response technician, a medical emergency technician (which is one with which I was particularly familiar) or a rescue squad man? How did the EMT relate at that point in time with the person who held the ultimate job, if you will, in the ambulance service — the ambulance driver? There was also a problem at the time with the acceptance of the paramedic. What was a paramedic? Not only did the individual himself or herself have somewhat of an identity crisis, but there was also some rampant paranoia among other health career professionals as to the role, responsibility and definition of a

Chris Gentile, Director, Office of Emergency Medical Services, Department of Health Services, Hartford, Conn.

paramedic. Additionally, we had a problem with semantics: "Paramedic, mobile intensive care technician, mobile intensive care unit technician, mobile intensive care paramedic, advanced EMT" — just what was this thing, the paramedic? We had to deal with the progression of emergency medical services from the ambulance service or the rescue squad into what we know today as the sophistication of an emergency medical services system.

Where are we? How far have we come? I think there is no real problem with the acceptance of the fact that the EMT is the grass roots provider of emergency health care in the streets, the cities and the roads of this country or wherever. The EMT has become a symbol, if you will. "EMT" is a household word.

Ironically, when one goes into some rural areas, the EMT today actually holds more prestige than many other professionals in the community. Coming from North Carolina, I can speak categorically of EMTs who are held in higher esteem in their communities than, in some cases, mayors, lawyers and many other professionals.

Training must be established now, not simply on an hourly designation, but based upon cognitive and manipulative competencies for the job that is defined. Although it has received some acclaim and some criticism, I recently wrote an article entitled, "The 81-Hour EMT Is Dead," and I think this is true because we can no longer subject ourselves to a time criterion. We know what the job description is for a basic level EMT. In fact, we should be more concerned about how do we meet that criterion, as opposed to how many hours we spend in class.

Training must move into the academic entities, the legitimate areas of learning, within our communities. I am not suggesting by this that they should be restricted to the college campus or the junior college or the community college or the technical institute or any other type of educational structure, but they must come under the aegis of the educational entity within the community or state. Certainly, hospital alliances must be sustained. They must be maintained for the clinical experience and exposure and for the determination of some practical competencies.

As we look at the EMT-Paramedic, we must recognize that for some time to come there will probably be the necessity for the home-grown programs, the programs geared specifically to a locality to generate a street level individual with the competencies of a paramedic. But that program, too, must move into the academic environment. Again, hospital relationships must be maintained. Training must come into a focus of compliance with the national standards for both EMT and EMT-P programs.

Why must this happen at this point in time in the EMS development? Simply put, the reason is to afford the professional an opportunity for career mobility. From this point on, and without any false interpretation, I am going to deal with the paid emergency medical services personnel. I say paid, as opposed to professional, because I know many volunteers who are just as professional in the carrying out of their EMS responsibilities as are those individuals who are paid. In no way am I trying to downgrade the importance of the volunteer EMT. However, when we talk in terms of careers, we are talking in terms of people who receive remuneration for their services and who are looking for higher rungs up the ladder of success to attain higher paying jobs.

As I foresee this career development and the inception of the training programs into the academic institutions, I see an evolution much like nursing has recently experienced. I see the EMT program coming at a certificate level, so that at the conclusion of that program, an individual has the credentials to enter a profession at the grass roots level. But the individual is given credit for that training, that education, so that that credit can be transferred to what should be an associate degree program, an associate of science in emergency medical science. This two-year program would give the individual street level competencies of an EMT-P. Additionally, it would give that individual a great deal more. A side benefit of the capabilities for the individual are the capabilities for the system. I said that we must maintain our local home-grown programs to meet immediate needs. But those programs are not going to be able to sustain themselves financially or in terms of teaching manpower to meet the ongoing replacement needs for EMS personnel. At that point, the only situation we need to address is the turnover. The associate degree level program can satisfy that need and also provide the individual a great degree more mobility.

What happens to this individual? With the associate degree programs, they are better qualified to move into supervisory roles. Once they have gained experience, we see them move into crew chief, shift superintendent, assistant director of local systems positions, etc. So the capability is there to move up on the EMS ladder in an organized career progression.

By the same token, though, we can look at some of the experiences since the 1970s; we recognize that, especially at the paramedic level, these people are burning out. They are fed up with the pressure of the constant life and death situation in the streets, the frustration of the back end of the unit. We are losing these people to other areas of public service. We are losing them to other health careers.

EMT-Ps have taken a certain period of time, be it five or six years, and during this time they have gained experience and training which is lost to today's EMS system because the individual is discouraged and is quitting. With a candidate who holds an associate degree, we have some alternatives for that person to keep him in the EMS system. When they are ready to move, I see several options open to them.

I see the option of patient care remaining open, so that once they want to be out of the field, once they want to be off the streets, again, educational opportunities are open to them to allow them to remain in patient care areas. I cite the entrance criteria for many physician's assistant training programs as two years of post high school education and at least 1,000 hours of patient contact. The associate degree EMT-P has met that requirement. A pilot program is underway right now in one particular state. The training program is intended to meet the staffing deficiencies of some of the small community rural hospitals which cannot today and which will never be able to afford full-time physician coverage.

If the individual is not interested in continuing patient care, what then? We must provide alternatives in career movement for that person as well. Again, the mechanisms have already been established in some states to accept the associate degree EMT-P for acceptance at a baccalaureate institution at the junior year and bring to that person academic skills in administration through education, so that he can assume positions of high administrative posts in EMS.

I consider myself to be very fortunate in that I have progressed nicely up the EMS ladder, but 90% of that was probably luck. Where do we get our training today as EMS administrators? The courses are just now beginning to emerge. I know of only about four institutions which offer degrees in EMS. The rest of us have all obtained our knowledge through hard knocks, coming up through the street. So this gives us an avenue of moving into administration. Perhaps an individual is interested in EMS education. By moving up to the baccalaureate institution, getting the appropriate education courses, that career goal can be satisfied.

I think there are two facts we must recognize in the development of career capability. As in any industry or profession, those who move up are going to be the cream of the crop. Second, those who move up are individuals who set their goals and took the necessary steps which were appropriate to achieving those goals so they would get to where they want to be. It is not the individual who sits back and says, "I am a paramedic. Being a paramedic now qualifies me to move up." That is not the case any longer. If one's goal is advanced patient care, set that goal and find out where your alternatives are and how you can apply some of the alternatives to get to where you want to be. If it is administration, look around for the applicability of using some of the educational opportunities you have had toward an administrative degree.

Self-Evaluation Quiz

1. We began to train EMTs in:
   a) 1850
   b) 1900
   c) 1950
   d) 1960
2. The EMT never really fit into the rural picture.
   a) True
   b) False
3. Paid emergency medical services personnel are:
   a) More reliable than volunteers
   b) Less reliable than volunteers
   c) Concerned eventually with higher paying jobs
   d) Discriminated against by volunteers

4. The author has experience with EMTs in:
   a) Anchorage, Alaska
   b) Birmingham, Alabama
   c) North Carolina
   d) Arkansas
5. Local "home-grown" EMT programs:
   a) Are out of the question
   b) Are here to stay
   c) Can help provisionally
   d) Do not exist for EMTs
6. The EMT can be compared with:
   a) An ambulance driver
   b) A fireman
   c) A nurse's aide
   d) An intern (physician)
   e) None of the above
7. EMT is certainly:
   a) No household word but still understood
   b) A household word
   c) No longer a concept for anyone
   d) Strictly for volunteers now

Answers on page 289.

Panel: EMT-Paramedic Training Programs

Alan Dimick, M.D.
Norman E. McSwain, Jr., M.D.
Charles Aprahamian, M.D.
Chris Gentile

Introduction

Alan Dimick, M.D.

As in any attempt to improve training and education at any level for the provision of medical care, the training of the personnel is extremely important. In this presentation we will discuss the training of EMTs and EMT-Paramedics. Many problems have been encountered in the development and organization of these programs, and Drs. McSwain, Aprahamian and Mr. Gentile will attempt to identify some of the more common problems and their solutions. These panel members have been involved in EMT and EMT-Paramedic training programs for many years and have encountered many problems which they will share with us. In particular they will discuss how these problems were resolved.

Because it is a medical care program, each training program must have a medical director, who will assist in the organization and development of the medical aspects of the training program as well as solve problems for it as time progresses. The program also needs an administrator to carry out the administrative aspects of the program as well as to construct the relationships with the parent educational institution for appropriate academic credits. Obviously the faculty must be composed of physicians, nurses, EMTs, pharmacists and other health care personnel. Classroom facilities are required for didactic as well as laboratory exercises. Equipment must be provided to the training program and dedicated to it. The training program cannot exist on equipment which is borrowed from other programs. An adequate library of reference books and journals is essential.

Alan Dimick, M.D., Associate Professor of Surgery, University of Alabama Medical Center, Birmingham; Member, Board of Directors, American Trauma Society.

The medical director will assist in the development of relationships with the local county medical society, the state medical association and the local hospitals.

In summary, the authors will discuss the methods used to implement EMT-Paramedic training programs in various areas throughout the nation and will share their problems as well as their successes.

Steps in Organizing and Establishing a Paramedic Training Program

Norman E. McSwain, Jr., M.D.

Objectives

To gain knowledge of the accreditation mechanism and training programs for EMT-Ps and insight into the bases of their effectiveness in serving the community.

Of all the elements required to organize the EMS training system program, the most important is the involvement of your local medical society. Without the close cooperation and early involvement of the local medical society, they will be against you. The local medical society is one organization which should be working for the program and their cooperation is paramount for success. You do not want to try to convince the medical society after the fact.

In developing a training program, particularly at the paramedic level, there is one thing of which you need to be aware. The American Medical Association is developing accreditation of training programs in the near future. Just as the AMA is accrediting other programs, such as the physicians assistant program, the surgical assistant program, respiratory therapy, medical technicians, cytology, x-ray technicians, it will soon accredit EMT-P programs.

In order to become accredited by the AMA accreditation system, one must have a well-organized system with a program that conforms to the National Curriculum objectives. In addition, it must be associated with an academic institution of some kind or at least some sort of mechanism whereby the

---

Norman E. McSwain, Jr., M.D., Associate Professor of Surgery, Tulane University School of Medicine, New Orleans, La.; Member, Board of Directors, American Trauma Society.

students can obtain classroom training, have audiovisuals and other teaching aspects.

There must be a medical director who is associated closely enough with the program so that he has program lecture and material approval, as well as objective approval. The medical director also must participate closely with the affiliated hospital so that the clinical experience is appropriate and the students get to accomplish in the hospital what in fact they should. He should then be affiliated closely with the services providing field internship.

In addition to the medical director, there must be a program director, whose responsibility is to set up the training program, based upon the standards. The program director may also be the medical director, but it works best if they are separate individuals. The program director's job is a full-time position, or at least the lead instructor's job is a full-time position, if the lead instructor is not the program director. It is very difficult to run an EMT-P training program with a half-time nurse or a third-time nurse spending a little bit of her time in her involvement. The nurse must prepare lectures and sit in on all of the lectures given by the other lecturers to see that the material is covered appropriately.

Additionally, there needs to be a standard mechanism of getting students in and out of a program, attending class, making sure that the class records are appropriate, making sure that the students have appeal procedures. The students must be evaluated prior to their admission, and the evaluation process must follow nondiscriminatory guidelines — those various functions that one would expect of any collegiate or noncollegiate institution.

After one completes a training program, it is appropriate to make application to the American Medical Association. The application will be done first by letter of intent which will be utilized to determine when the site evaluation will occur. Then, at some future time, probably three months prior to the on-site evaluation, the application form will be due.

The application form is in itself an in-depth evaluation of the training program because it allows for information by the program itself. It is almost a self-evaluation form, noting the particular strengths and weaknesses of the individual training program.

After the application is completed (it will take approximately 20 man-hours to complete the application), it is sent to the National Association of Emergency Medical Technicians (administrating organization for the accreditation). The application will be referred to those individuals who comprise the on-site evaluation team.

The on-site evaluation team will be composed of three individuals who will spend approximately two days at the site. The accreditation will probably be for a four-year period with on-site evaluations at the end of each four-year period. The joint review committee will be sponsored by six organizations: the American College of Surgeons, the American College of Emergency Physicians, the American Psychiatric Association, the American Society of Anesthesiologists, the National Association of Emergency Medical Technicians and the National Registry of Emergency Medical Technicians.

The on-site evaluations will be referred back to the joint review committee, which will review the applications and the recommendations of the on-site evaluators. Then the final judgments for accreditation and what type of accreditation, whether it will be one-year accreditation because of some weaknesses in the program or a total four-year approval, are made.

Does every community need a paramedic program? If they do not have enough patients to maintain their skills, or if they do not have enough in-service training to maintain their skills, they should be functioning as an EMT intermediate, and that is an EMT who can place IVs and Esophageal Obturator Airway after appropriately assessing the patient's problem. I say this, realizing that there is an EMT-P program in Kansas, where there is a community of 10,000, which is functioning well and has 37% of their overall on-the-scene defibrillations go home from the hospital alive. This is without medical communication to the hospital. They are functioning entirely on standing orders. That violates many rules that are held sacred. But there is one thing about this system that makes it different from any of the rest. Every morning they have a one- to two-hour station drill for a cardiac arrest 365 days a year. If there is that kind of dedication to continuing education and skill maintenance, it can be done in a small community. But if the attitude is "Well, simply wait until there is an ambulance run and the cardiac arrest victim to gain skills," then it will not work.

There is a good reason that community colleges have absolutely no business in the training of EMTs. They are interested in turning out numbers and they do not care about job opportunities and how many of these graduates will have an opportunity to go to work. Devote one or two schools or more if approved in the entire state to training the EMT-Ps and then those must have a three-year or a five-year limit, and when the job opportunities in the state are filled, close the program down.

Dr. Chan Hering and I think basically the same way about accreditation. I lean toward some national organization doing it because we do not want to turn out a population of people who can just work from one border of the state to the other. We want to train individuals who have career opportunities to move from Florida to California to Kansas to Missouri. I think some national organization should set standards and people should follow them, both in the accreditation of training programs and the certification of the qualifications of the individual.

Self-Evaluation Quiz

1. The local medical society:
   a) Has nothing to do with EMTs
   b) Must get involved in EMT programs early
   c) Is the worst enemy of EMTs
   d) Can only become involved with EMT programs late on in their existence, not at the beginning
2. According to the author, all community colleges should not train EMTs.
   a) True
   b) False
3. An EMT program:
   a) Should not have to conform to National Curriculum objectives
   b) Should have to conform
   c) Should not have to conform if an M.D. directs the program
   d) Is automatically accredited by the AMA

4. How many people perform a site evaluation?
   a) None. It is only simulated.
   b) 2
   c) 3
5. Accreditation will most likely be for:
   a) 2 years
   b) 3 years
   c) 4 years
   d) 5 years
6. The joint review committee is composed of how many organizations?
   a) 3
   b) 4
   c) 5
   d) 6
7. Accreditation might be for only one year if:
   a) The American College of Surgeons is absent from the joint committee
   b) The American Psychiatric Association is absent
   c) Some weaknesses are spotted in the EMT program
   d) The on-site evaluation takes only two days

Answers on page 289.

Statewide Design of a Paramedic System: The Wisconsin Approach

Charles Aprahamian, M.D.

Objectives

1. To define a paramedic in terms of his terminal behavior.
2. To discuss the training programs needed to achieve that level.
3. To discuss the selection of trainees.
4. To discuss the testing of the finished product.
5. To discuss licensure of the paramedic so that he can function.

Wisconsin addressed the issues of paramedics in 1973 – the year enabling legislation was passed for the Regulation of EMT-Basic and EMT-Advanced personnel. This legislation addressed the capabilities, training, testing, licensing and the provision of services.

As to his capabilities, the EMT-Paramedic was defined as an emergency medical technician with certain "plus" attributes. The terminal behavior was identifed in the statutes as the ability to (1) give parenteral medication, (2) initiate intravenous fluids, (3) insert nasogastric tubes, (4) pass endotracheal tubes and (5) apply electroshock to a pulseless nonbreathing victim.

To achieve these stated objectives, a curriculum was sought, and in the absence of a national standard, the two Wisconsin medical schools' paramedic programs submitted theirs, and a composite served to approve others. The educational process revolved about didactic and manipulative skills and was followed by a period of supervised field experience. Recently, the paramedic curriculum's objectives were reviewed and it was

---

Charles Aprahamian, M.D., Assistant Professor of Surgery, Medical College of Wisconsin, Milwaukee.

noted that the two medical schools had a different number of hours. The Medical College of Wisconsin had approximately 1,000 hours in its curriculum, and the University of Wisconsin-Madison had 700 hours. In order to arrive at some acceptable standard throughout the state, the National Highway Traffic Safety Association (NHTSA) Paramedic Program is now being reviewed. At the moment, it would appear that the national standard is a maximum standard, and what Wisconsin is desirous of is a minimum standard. In many communities, we don't need or want all those skills taught and/or used. I believe Wisconsin is going to remove from the national curriculum those sections which are not needed, thereby extracting the critical essence of the course which will become Wisconsin's standard. If training centers want to use the maximum standards as listed in the NHTSA curriculum, so be it. But those who use the minimum standards, "the Wisconsin standard," will also be approved.

The testing for licensure took several years to develop and, in 1978, consisted of a written, practical and oral examination. Before entering the examination process, the training program medical director had to state that the applicant for licensure had satisfactorily completed the program and was sufficiently prepared for licensure. If the medical director certified the student and the applicant for licensure satisfactorily completed the written and practical examination, the oral exam became a perfunctory approval.

Wisconsin's EMT-Paramedic Licensure Regulations empowered the Division of Health to not only test and license the paramedic but to approve and license the EMS program in which the paramedic would function. These programs had to have some semblance of an EMS system with approved facilities, trained manpower, ambulance services, communications and an effort directed toward public information/education.

Once the paramedic is licensed, he can function only within the approved paramedic (EMS) system. If the paramedic were to leave the community (for example, on vacation), he could not function as a paramedic in his new locale but could provide basic EMT skills. If he chose to function as a paramedic and to administer advanced life support skills, he could be held liable for his actions. The intent of this mechanism was to assure that the trained paramedic could function only in an approved and licensed EMS service area.

In Wisconsin, there are approximately 10,000 EMTs, less than 2% of which are paramedics. They function within large communities. Only two of these communities have hospitals with areawide capabilities (Level I). It is interesting to note that in only one of the seven programs do the paramedics function only to provide paramedic skills as listed in the State statute. In the other six areas, the paramedic units function as primary response units and supplement advanced life support skills when needed.

The selection of the paramedic trainee is a function of the paramedic plan. The EMS Committee in Milwaukee decided that the fire service would be the responsible agency for providing paramedic care. Therefore, the only people who are to be trained by the "approved training center" in the Milwaukee area would be fire personnel. In another community, it was decided that half of the paramedic services would be fire personnel and the other half would be from private ambulances. On the whole, at least in Wisconsin, the majority of the personnel are from the fire service. If the community is responsible for providing the training and, hence, the financial obligation that goes with it, I think they will see to it that only a minimal number are trained, rather than just giving the responsibility of training to vocational technical institutes which, I believe, would basically want to train for the sake of training because the school's income is dependent upon that training. Another way of controlling the student population is to make sure that they work only in approved programs. If their ability to work depends upon a double licensure (portion of the license relates to the paramedic functioning as a paramedic, and the other half relates to the paramedic functioning in an approved licensed paramedic program), then what is the sense of graduating 250 paramedics per year if only ten are going to be able to work?

In Wisconsin, there are no paramedics in a volunteer service. Eighty percent of the EMTs in Wisconsin are in volunteer service, and we have only a few municipal, full-time fire departments which are readily involved in ambulance service. Paramedic services are basically out of the major fire departments in Wisconsin. We have no volunteers. Having said that, let me give two exceptions. In the Brown County area, which includes Green Bay, a portion of the paramedic services is provided by a volunteer ambulance force. We recently approved a paramedic training program in Door County, a nice vacation area which wanted to have paramedics. They maintained that they had a system that was viable and were going to use a volunteer force to provide the care. They seemed to think that they could put on the training so the State Training Committee approved their request, believing that it would be interesting to see what the result would be. Could they, in fact, produce a product that was worthwhile? If such a program would work, and they could prove it, then I think paramedics would be a viable force in a rural community. So we are looking to Door County with interest.

Self-Evaluation Quiz

1. A paramedic can be defined as being a basic EMT who has attained selected advanced life support skills.
   a) True
   b) False
2. A Wisconsin paramedic with training can provide his skills at any time and in any place.
   a) True
   b) False
3. The majority of EMTs in all states are paramedics.
   a) True
   b) False
4. In Wisconsin, the majority of the personnel providing paramedic services are within the fire service.
   a) True
   b) False
5. All paramedic programs should have equal number of hours of training.
   a) True
   b) False

Answers on page 289.

Quality Control in a Paramedic Program

Chris Gentile

Objectives

To become familiar with the context of professional paramedics, their training, certification and competencies.

The pitfalls of developing a paramedic program are relatively well known. Much of the impetus for the development of a paramedic program comes from the providers, especially in the rural areas, i.e., the volunteers. They want to be like their city counterparts and they want to be paramedics. This can create several problems and I think it is incumbent upon us not to let the provider organizations push us too quickly too soon. Clearly, we must identify some of the capabilities and arrange for some cooperation, not only of clinical facilities that surround the area, but also of all entities within the area that are in existence.

First, we must decide on the most appropriate organization or agency to provide the paramedic level of care, taking into consideration that there are several alternatives. Is the volunteer rescue squad in a rural community the most appropriate mechanism to provide paramedic service? Or, is it better to incorporate the transportation capability of the volunteers with a paramedic response out of another organization or entity, even quite possibly out of the hospital?

In the development of the program itself, we should analyze some ancillary or nonmedical resources, such as the educational institutions. Some parts of the country have a very widespread

Chris Gentile, Director, Office of Emergency Medical Services, Department of Health Services, Hartford, Conn.

capability in terms of academic institutions in our community, i.e., community college and technical institutes. These institutions can add valuable resources, not only in terms of facilities, but also in terms of manpower, by giving us some administrative support. We have already heard the necessity for having this. Additionally, they can provide some of the necessary teaching capability. This utilization can reduce the financial burden of paramedic training which is usually borne by the hospital itself. However, we cannot deny that the actual final medical responsibility rests within the clinical facility; experiential training under close medical supervision must take place in the hospital and encompass all clinical areas.

An area which I personally feel is often overlooked is the supervision of field performance prior to full certification. There are several methods of that field supervision, one of which comes as a result of direct physician observation and the other, with mobile intensive care nurses or some specially recognized nurses performing the supervision in the field. Peer review is also a customary mechanism for field performance review but is acceptable only when performed by experienced, mature paramedics. Unfortunately, I do not have any answer. Perhaps a combination of all three is best. I do think this is an area where we must take a serious look before we can give our stamp of approval to a paramedic training program.

Another pitfall we have identified is levels of competency. What happens, especially in the rural areas, with different EMS providers relating to one facility. How do we identify what the capability is of this particular ambulance service provider or paramedic provider? Often, we build into our systems a confusion factor by dissecting the paramedic training program into too many subprograms. We have an intravenous fluids level-capable individual, we have a cardiac technician, we have this and that specialist, and it becomes extremely confusing to the medical personnel on the hospital side of the two-way radio. I think this can lead not only to operational but to legal problems as well.

We are trying to strive for acceptance of paramedic training for college level credit for the sake of the paramedics and especially in the paid personnel area. We are seeing the establishment of some career tracks in emergency medical services and some of those tracks are based on academic credit. This is a must.

In terms of the areas that I see that must be addressed, there are two key people in the paramedic program, both in its initial implementation and on an ongoing basis. These have both already been identified for you. There must be a physician-director. We heard of the medical society's or the medical staff's involvement, but there must be one physician who is going to accept the responsibility of overall medical direction and control. Too many systems receive their medical direction from general input from the medical staff. We need one physician who can say, "This is my baby and I am going to spend the amount of necessary time to make sure it runs right." By the same token, we need that one administrative person who is going to make sure that all of the detail work is covered, all the necessary bases are touched, all the administrative people are informed and the hospital staffs are knowledgeable.

The most difficult point to address in the development of a paramedic program is where to draw the line in terms of cost effectiveness. How much is it going to cost? What are the chrome and plastic niceties we want on top, or do we just need a bare bones, basic life support system to really address the needs in terms of cost effectiveness?

Skill maintenance can be addressed by a solid ongoing continuing education program. This can be the answer for the small community where skills may not be maintained by actual performance. This is especially true in areas where you are dealing with volunteers and you do not have them locked in on a day-to-day basis for inhouse, inservice education.

Perhaps another solution to this type of problem (and somewhere along the line, someone is going to have to bite the bullet) is to say, "Look, rescue squad, we appreciate your dedication and we would like to incorporate you into our paramedic program but maybe you are not the providers of the paramedic care, but please help us as the transportation entity." The hospital perhaps — and I say this only as an alternative — can employ one or two paramedics on each shift, making sure that there are sufficient people to cover all shifts, to provide the paramedic capability out of the hospital, leaving the transportation and basic life support to the fire department rescue squad.

This boosts the ego of the rescue squad by incorporating them into the paramedic program and it still provides enough patient experience to a select few people at the paramedic level to keep their skills from deteriorating.

I think the community colleges and the vocational technical schools and institutes have a definite role. There are areas that address the open-door policy of the community colleges and technical institutes in virtually all states with which I am familiar and there are program criteria that allow you to have closed-door programs, that is, to set limits on enrollment, to set criteria for where these programs are going to be put on. It is necessary to recognize that a paramedic training program is not like a school for mechanics or welders. It is a special program with unique characteristics. You can close the doors of enrollment to the program. I support very strongly the fact that there has to be a limit on the number of persons trained and they must have places to go when they are trained. But the open-door criteria that the community colleges profess, by which they say they must let everybody in, is their own simple means of trying to pass the responsibility to somebody else. They have the capability to close their doors if they should want to do so.

With regard to a national accreditation or certification, the only way it will work from an administrative or a paramedic standpoint is if the organization, be it the American Medical Association or whatever, takes into account the fact that there are unique needs in different types of geographic areas and does not set the program standards so high that they are unobtainable for the rural communities or for the areas where recognition is needed, where the requirements sought are so far above the capabilities of that teaching facility. If we can recognize the intermediate levels of a paramedic, in such a manner that they gain the acceptance of a national organization, then it will work. If the program criteria for national recognition are so stringent that many of the rural states and rural communities cannot meet them, then the states are going to go their own way.

We have had some experience with volunteer paramedics. We have found that we kept the criteria for their certification the same. Along the lines that were just discussed, I think we must recognize that we are dealing with technicians. We are not dealing with independent practitioners. The reason why a paramedic will lose his certification or license or whatever the legalistic method for performance is in any particular state, when they leave that particular program, is because they are accountable back to the medical controls of that particular paramedic system. If they go into an area where there is no paramedic system, they do not have the medical controls. So I think it is incumbent that the certification, registration and licensure be dependent upon that affiliation. The same thing can apply to the volunteer. If the person moves from a paramedic volunteer system to another paramedic volunteer system that fits the criteria and is accepted by the medical controls of that particular system, there is no reason why he cannot function. But if he moves to an area where the system is not developed, he literally cannot function.

With regard to insurance, the municipal or governmental employees do have insurance available to them. I know of only one insurer who is writing paramedic insurance and it is only to the intermediate level, including IV and esophageal obturator airway, and that is a company headquartered in New York. After fairly exhaustive research, it is the only one we have found which will write a private operator or a volunteer rescue squad for any kind of paramedic coverage.

Self-Evaluation Quiz

1. According to the author, the hidden problems of a paramedic program are yet to be uncovered.
   a) True
   b) False
2. Rural volunteer medical workers:
   a) Do not exist
   b) Want to emulate their city counterparts
   c) Should all be paid
3. Peer review by paramedics:
   a) Is impossible
   b) Is best done by idealistic younger members
   c) Is best done by experienced mature paramedics
   d) Should be done quarterly

4. We want:
   a) Acceptance of paramedic training for college-level credit
   b) High-school-level training for paramedics
   c) None of the above
5. Cost effectiveness:
   a) Is not involved in paramedic programs
   b) Is a difficult aspect of paramedic programs
   c) Is involved, but only peripherally, with paramedic programs
   d) Concerns M.D.s but not EMT-Ps
6. We must:
   a) Never give rescue squads the impression that they can't be paramedics
   b) Dispose completely of rescue squads
   c) Pay all volunteer rescue squads (so we can then fire them)
   d) Gently convert rescue squads to transport units, if need be
7. Paramedic training must be on an open-door basis, with the opportunity for any interested person to try his or her hand at helping the community.
   a) True
   b) False
8. How many insurers write paramedic insurance?
   a) None
   b) 1
   c) 4
   d) 5
9. The supervision of field performance prior to full certification is:
   a) Well organized and at an ideal level
   b) Inapplicable to parametic training and activity
   c) Often overlooked
   d) None of the above
10. Levels of competency:
    a) Are the perfect solution to differing abilities
    b) Give the hospital side of the two-way radio assurance that a patient is in good hands
    c) Confuse the patient
    d) Confuse the medical personnel on the hospital side of the radio

Answers on page 289.

Development of Transfer and Triage Protocols

Paul R. Meyer, Jr., M.D.

Objectives

1. To introduce the concept of a multistate spine center and to examine the transfer agreements and protocols for providing early identification of trauma and improved care, including rehabilitation of victims.
2. To consider a typical transfer protocol.
3. To review statistical results (retrieval and admission) of the Spine Center at Northwestern Memorial Hospital.

Spinal cord injury is one of three major areas of trauma where a significant effort is being made to provide for early injury identification and improved care. Now in its seventh year of federal sponsorship, the spine injury program at Northwestern University retrieves patients from a five-state area, utilizing the Illinois Trauma System. The catchment area which is affected by this Center contains a population of 20 million people, coming from the states of Indiana, Michigan, Ohio, Wisconsin, Iowa and Illinois.

In 1974, a brochure on the reasons, needs and accessibility of spine-injured patients to the Spinal Injury Center was developed and mailed to every emergency room in the five-state area defined above. A phone number was provided, with the assurance that if the injury was identified, regardless of the distance, the Spine Center would initiate care, retrieve the patient and provide total care, including rehabilitation and vocational reeducation. The response was so effective that it

---

Paul R. Meyer, Jr., M.D., Co-Director, Midwest Regional Spinal Cord Injury Care System, Northwestern Memorial Hospital, Chicago, Ill.

became imperative that a triage and transfer protocol be developed.

Dr. David Boyd, Director of Emergency Medical Services, Department of Health, Education and Welfare, has urged over the past four years that transfer agreements and protocols be developed between participating institutions. It is not easily done. First, it is not easy to establish a recognized and utilized regional facility, supposedly more capable in one area of trauma management than all of the other facilities in your immediate area. As an example, within Chicago, there are more than 100 hospitals with emergency rooms, yet there are now only three recognized comprehensive medical-trauma facilities or institutions with voice communication and medical control of the ambulances operating within the metropolitan Chicago area. These three institutions are also responsible for advanced life support continuing education and to be centers of excellence in comprehensive medical-trauma care 24 hours a day. Northwestern Memorial Hospital is one of the three described institutions with a general medical-trauma hospital, a woman's and psychiatric hospital, a rehabilitation hospital and a veteran hospital within the complex. Thus, patients from each category would be eligible for transfer to this Center. In particular and as referenced in the data being presented, the principal trauma program at Northwestern was the Acute Spinal Injury Center. In concept, therefore, a transfer protocol takes into account what it is you have to offer, how you propose to retrieve your population and how you wish to initiate the care process.

It is important to understand the Illinois Trauma Program organization, or that of any state, when developing the instruments to be used in the development of intrahospital transfer agreements and protocols. For example, for every trauma center in Illinois, there is an assigned trauma coordinator — or a total of 49 trauma coordinators. The primary responsibility of the coordinator assigned to Northwestern is the transfer to the institution of spinal cord injuries from a five-state area and pediatric emergencies throughout a similar area. The way a transfer is effected is as follows: A trauma coordinator in the field identifies the presence of a particular injury which has been retrieved and brought to one of the local or area trauma facilities. All patients are first taken to an initial care trauma facility. Thus, the initial treating hospital becomes the "*referring*" institution and the tertiary or comprehensive institution becomes the "*receiving*" institution.

In the absence of a formal written transfer agreement, the state trauma program serves as the instrument for the transfer, and the qualifications for transfer are established within.

As an example of the mechanism utilized for transfer of a patient, let us identify the patient as a spinal cord injury victim. The trauma coordinator assigned to the referring institution contacts the trauma coordinator assigned to the Spinal Cord Injury Center. In turn, he notifies the responsible physician to whom the patient will be assigned. The two physicians (referring and receiving) communicate and agree to transfer the patient. The trauma coordinator assumes responsibility for obtaining the appropriate mode of transportation and notifies the receiving hospital of the patient's estimated time of arrival (ETA). At the same time, the physician to be responsible for the patient's care notifies the trauma team and emergency room of the patient's diagnosis, the problems related to the patient's transfer, the recommended management techniques to be performed prior to the patient's transfer (blood administration, tracheostomy). All this having been performed — the patient identified, the trauma coordinator notified, the receiving physician notified, the trauma team and hospital alerted — the patient is transferred with a known ETA.

Possibly not in all instances in general trauma, but definitely in spine and neurological trauma, it is important that no patient in the field be transferred directly to a comprehensive hospital without evaluation first in a primary care hospital. This is particularly true for a patient with multiple system injuries, who is to be transported over a long distance. If, for any reason, the patient does not fall into a category of a safe and manageable transfer, the patient should not be transferred at all. That is a decision for physicians to make simultaneously from both ends. Appropriate care procedure is then instituted which will allow for transfer when various requirements have been met. Thus, the transfer protocol is instituted.

Transfer Protocol

The protocol for the spine injured patient may not be the same as that for burns, poisons, behavioral or neonatal emergencies, yet they are specific for the entity.

1. Upon notification of a spine injury referral, referring physician-receiving physician contact is made where indicated.
2. If the patient is a cervical spine injury, the following are requested:
   a) Baseline arterial blood gases
   b) Intravenous fluids
   c) Urinary catheter
   d) Nasogastric tube
   e) Administration of dexamethasone 20 mg IV push and mannitol 500 cc - 20% to run over two hours
   f) Nasal oxygen during transfer
   g) Appropriate spine splinting (spineboard or Orthosis)
   h) All cervical spine patients should be accompanied by a trained ICU, trauma nurse or respiratory therapist.
   i) All hospital records and x-rays must accompany the patient's transfer.
   j) We will anticipate the arrival of the patient by notifying specific consultants:
      1. The emergency room and Spinal Cord Unit.
      2. Orthopedic and neurosurgery residents and staff on call.
      3. Anesthesia and respiratory therapy on all quadriplegics and upper thoracic injuries (to evaluate in the ER).
      4. General surgery on all multitrauma victims.

By way of explanation, the value of the nasogastric tube is in the prevention of, or reduction of, abdominal distention. Several events occur with distention: vomiting with possible aspiration and restriction of already compromised diaphragmatic excursion due to bowel distention in the quadriplegic. Likewise, due to the presence of compromised respiration in the quadriplegic, during transfer, oxygen should be administered and the aircraft kept either below 8,000 feet, or the transfer done in a pressurized aircraft. Obtaining arterial gases (on room air) prior to patient transfer allows for immediate "trending" with the obtaining of similar studies on arrival. Thus, the need for referring hospital records and x-rays.

It should be stated that a physician is seldom required for transport of a spine injured patient unless the patient's life is threatened. This more often occurs in the patient with a cervical spine injury above C-5 (where the phrenic nerves may become involved) or with the multitrauma patient.

Conclusions

Try never to transfer a patient between two institutions without physician-to-physician knowledge. The above transfer protocol procedures have been developed by time and situation testing over a seven-year period. Fulfilling each area mentioned leaves little to be required of or questioned when the patient arrives and has been of immeasurable assistance in improving and smoothing out patient transfers and patient care.

The Illinois Trauma System and the Spinal Injury System have been in operation for about seven years. Recently, an out-of-state hospital initiated on their own a written transfer agreement with the Spinal Injury Center. Heretofore, the agreement was a referral through and by means of the Illinois Trauma System and a verbal acceptance of the spine trauma patient by the Spine Center. Inasmuch as the Spine Center received patients from a five-state area (having greater than 700 hospitals), it would be impossible to obtain a written agreement with each. On the other hand, we now have an independent hospital in another state sending us a written transfer protocol for approval. It is interpreted to mean that the hospitals in the field are beginning to recognize (a) there is a system by which they can transfer patients up the line and (b) medicolegally, there are disease entities which require transfer for more sophisticated care. Thus, a need for a written transfer agreement.

Obviously, what we are striving for, using the transfer agreement as the vehicle, is a smoothing out of the care process. That is coming to the forefront and is the reason why hospitals must implement transfer agreements. By establishing a transfer agreement at the administrative level (the chief of staff and the hospital administrator), it becomes possible to circumvent the physician who refuses to participate appropriately. The hospital administration then can identify those physicians who are not cooperating. I think time will change the complacency and reluctance which exists in some areas. Just to carry that one step further, once the patient enters your hospital and is transferred to another institution, that other institution, regardless of the advice, suggestions and help they may have contributed to a patient's transfer, is not medicolegally responsible for that patient until he enters your hospital's back door. The referring hospital is responsible up to that time.

The Spine Center at Northwestern will accept the acutely injured patient at any time, but we strive for arrival within four hours of injury. In the past three years, we have retrieved 26% of our patients in the first 4 hours, 61% in 6 hours and 94% in 24 hours, with a mean admission time of 8.6 hours. Appreciating that this mean admission time includes trauma, primary care hospital, air transportation cross-country and arrival at Spine Center, a lapsed time of 8.6 hours is quite remarkable.

Self-Evaluation Quiz

1. A physician is seldom required for transport of a spine injured patient unless the patient's life is threatened.
   a) True
   b) False
2. In spine and neurological trauma, no patient in the field should be transferred directly to a comprehensive hospital without evaluation in a primary care hospital.
   a) True
   b) False
3. Cervical injured patients receive:
   a) Dexamethasone 30 mg IV and mannitol 500 cc 20%
   b) Dexamethasone 20 mg IV and mannitol 250 cc 20%
   c) Dexamethasone 20 mg IV and mannitol 500 cc 40%
   d) Dexamethasone 20 mg IV and mannitol 500 cc 20%
4. What is the mean admission time (lapsed time) for patients reaching the Spine Center at Northwestern Memorial?
   a) 4.6 hours
   b) 6.5 hours
   c) 8.6 hours
   d) 9.2 hours

5. What patients should be accompanied by a trained ICU, trauma nurse or respiratory specialist?
   a) Femur injuries
   b) Thoracic injuries
   c) Cervical injuries
   d) Gut injuries

Answers on page 289.

Categorization: Definitions and Rationale

John W. Otten, M.D.

Objectives

1. To describe a categorization process as it was implemented in Region 1-B, State of Illinois in 1971.
2. To show that this gradual transition of response capabilities to meet the needs of the critically ill and injured is not only cost effective but does not initiate a marked change in the normal physician-patient relationship or physician referral patterns.
3. To show that the systems approach to the care of the critically injured is also capable of reducing mortality from serious injuries.

Current high costs of the delivery of medical services mandate that a more cost-effective solution to medical problems be found. The categorization of hospitals is the most cost-effective way to insure maximum patient care for Emergency Medical Services (EMS). In 1970 Dr. David Boyd and then Governor Richard B. Ogilvie implemented what was then known as the State of Illinois Trauma Program. The Program began in 1971 and it is of interest that in 1976 the *Bulletin of the American College of Surgeons* reported on the task force of the Committee on Trauma and its decisions on the categorization of hospitals for EMS. It states that the responsibility for providing optimum hospital resources for the care of the seriously injured rests inescapably with hospital trustees, administrators, physicians and nurses. There is probably no single term that elicits the anxiety reaction more than the word

---

John W. Otten, M.D., Medical Director, Regional Trauma Center, St. Francis Hospital Medical Center, Peoria, Ill.; Founding Member, American Trauma Society.

categorization. Physicians who have been friends for many years, although they might be competitors, turn from reasonable men into aggressive antagonists. The rationality that we normally associate with physicians and administrators changes and changes dramatically. I seriously doubt that this panic reaction is really justified. Are all of our pontifical statements on categorization destroying physician-patient relationships, infringing upon private practice, decreasing the hospital bed census? Are all of these fears really justified? What is this new bureaucratic monster that Dr. David Boyd has encouraged to be developed throughout the United States?

First, it might be a surprise that it is not new. The October 1968 issue of the *Bulletin of the American College of Surgeons* contains an article by the late Dr. Oscar Hampton who is considered by many to be the father of the present day approach to the trauma problem. Dr. Hampton was highly respected by everyone because of his approach and his concern for the critically ill and injured. In this article, statements were made which were prophetic.

Dr. Hampton listed eight criteria for an optimum EMS system. Among these were standardization of ambulance design and logistical placement of ambulances, central dispatch of emergency vehicles, trained attendants manning these vehicles, standardized equipment, two-way radio contact with hospitals, fully equipped emergency rooms manned 24 hours a day, exchange of expensive equipment and standardized record-keeping. He stressed the need for a systemized approach to the care of the critically injured. He went on to state that "those emergency departments which cannot meet the standards set forth by the American College of Surgeons or those to be issued in the future by the joint commission should be closed." In 1971 the American Medical Association published the guidelines for the categorization of hospital emergency departments.

It is rather interesting that some of the pioneers in the care of trauma patients realized that once the patient arrived at their institution, the patient would probably not receive good care and many of them would not survive. Among these pioneers were Drs. Alan Dimick, Curtis Artz, Deke Farrington who wrote the famous article, "Death in the Ditch," Charles Fitz, Charles Frey who has been and still is very active in the College of

Surgeons, Dr. Oscar Hampton, Dr. Gene Nagel and Cuthbert Owens of Denver. They met under the auspices of the American Medical Association and issued several statements.

In the preamble to this article they stated that the basic purpose of categorization is to "identify the readiness and capability of a hospital and its entire staff to receive and treat correctly and expeditiously the emergent patients." This statement was made not in 1976 or 1977, but in 1971. It further stated that a total categorization of a hospital's capabilities may evolve so that selected hospitals might close, in fact, *should* close their emergency departments, thus conserving resources and money while other hospitals will expand their capabilities to treat the emergent patient. Again, this was in 1971 before high medical cost was a number one priority of an economy-conscious administration. Among the participating organizations that sponsored this task force was the American College of Surgeons Committee on Trauma, The Committee on Injuries of the American Academy of Orthopedic Surgeons, the Arlie Conference of Emergency Medical Services and the American Medical Association.

Returning to the more recent article — the September 1976 *Bulletin of the American College of Surgeons* — it states that "hospital resources for the care of the seriously injured are not optimal unless they include clearly defined relationships and prearranged transfer plans between referring physicians and hospitals." A trauma service must be a multidisciplinary service, headed by a surgeon with a separate ICU and priority access to all of the facilities within the hospital such as the radiology department and the laboratory.

The guidelines for the categorization in this particular article classified hospitals into three groups based upon levels of care capabilities. It is interesting to note that this categorization plan is very similar to that of the categorization plan adopted previously by Illinois.

The optimum criteria, according to the College of Surgeons, must include 24-hour inhouse presence of all surgical specialties and subspecialties, inhouse anesthesia service, cardiologist, internal medicine, pediatrics, blood bank, nuclear medicine, diagnostic radiologist, angiography, dialysis capabilities and, of course, immediate access to the OR and to the ICUs.

The intermediate hospital does not have to be quite so sophisticated, but it does require quite the same inhouse personnel to respond to emergencies. The minimal standards deal primarily with the less severely injured or if a critically injured individual is brought to the institution, resuscitation, stabilization and preparation for transfer to another facility must be within the realm of the capabilities of this minimal institution.

In July 1978 a joint meeting on classification was held by the American Hospital Association and the American Medical Association. This meeting, by invitation only, represented a broad cross-section of individuals throughout the United States involved with Emergency Medicine. This two-day workshop divided participants into seven critical areas as outlined in the federal guidelines. In addition, workshops were conducted in other areas such as transfer agreements, medical control and how the entire plan related to the categorization of facilities. The preliminary results of that meeting will be published in December 1979, but it is anticipated that there will be no drastic changes from that outlined by the American College of Surgeons.

Recently, an article in the *Journal of Emergency Medical Services* referred to the joint commission on hospital accreditation. According to that article beginning in January 1979, hospitals seeking accreditation from the joint commission will be evaluated for compliance with the newly revised standards for emergency services. They do not say who is going to establish those standards. It is somewhat disconcerting when one further learns from this article that four levels of recommended hospital response capabilities are to be recommended rather than the three as previously mentioned.

With this background information I think that it is appropriate to relate our experience in what I would consider a typical midwestern city in which there were three hospitals. Each of these three hospitals maintained an ER and attempted to provide 24-hour service to respond to all types of emergencies. When the categorization process was implemented in Illinois and the designation of trauma centers occurred, one of the great advantages that we had was that we did not know exactly what was happening. Occasionally being in the dark can be advantageous. At an executive committee meeting our administrator very happily announced that we had been designated as a trauma center. Our response was: "That is fine. What is a trauma center?" At the next surgical department meeting we invited our administrator to attend and asked him some very pointed questions. Very honestly, the surgical staff at St. Francis Hospital was extremely upset because no one had consulted them regarding their involvement in such a system. Having a teaching program, residents, an obligation to teach these residents and medical school affiliation, we were certain that we were doing an adequate job in handling the critically injured patients. We also felt that we had a sufficient patient load of trauma to teach our medical students and our house staff effectively to care for these patients. Our concerns were that a large percentage of the trauma cases are the unfortunate ones in any given community. They are the alcoholics, the police characters. They get into fights and there are shootings and stabbings. Although this does provide teaching material, it is very time-consuming for the attending staff. It was our concern, and more appropriately it was actually a panic reaction among the surgical staff at St. Francis Hospital, that we would be in our ER night after night ministering to all of the unfortunates in the entire region rather than our own city. This, however, has not materialized. The majority of the patients transferred to us are accident victims. Another rather interesting aspect of this transfer pattern is that 78% of the people transferred to us are covered by insurance, 3.9% are public aid or clinic-type patients and the remainder pay the bill themselves. This refutes the statement of many physicians that their institutions would become "a dumping ground" in such a system.

The public image on the other hand were the very visible signs that were erected around Illinois directing people to the "trauma centers." These signs not only prompted much concern among those hospitals not so designated but provided ambulance drivers from out of town direct access in unfamiliar surroundings to a trauma center. The public, on the other hand, became more aware that a system had been implemented to provide them with adequate care in catastrophic situations.

One of the concerns of institutions that are discussing the categorization concept is that no institution within a particular designation region may fulfill all of the requirements to be designated as a regional trauma center. In a situation such as this, the categorization process is flexible enough to allow for certain deficiencies. If these deficient areas can be met by a systematic, rapid transfer mechanism, this will be acceptable. For example, even though St. Francis Hospital, a regional center, is an 840-bed hospital we do not have a burn center. Therefore, we were required to provide a burn center care program and we accomplished this by utilization of the Illinois Department of Transportation helicopters to transfer the patients to the burn center after stabilization and resuscitation at our institution. Other of the critical care areas mandated by the federal government such as poison control, neonatal, cardiac, spinal cord injury and psychiatric emergencies were provided by our institution. As the concept developed in Region 1-B we began to see patients more frequently arriving at our institution that we were convinced would never have survived if it were not for the system. Our institution began to receive more and more patients in a stable condition; the other institutions within Peoria were receiving fewer critical patients. Nurses at Methodist Hospital began applying for positions at St. Francis Hospital. We also heard that some of the surgeons at Methodist and Proctor hospitals were unhappy because they were not included in the trauma surgery due to the categorization and the designation of St. Francis Hospital as the center. What then occurred was that a number of those surgeons applied and were given privileges at our institution and to take call on our trauma roster.

If one considers it from a practical standpoint, however, three hospitals in a community of approximately 250,000 population cannot provide three ERs capable of responding to the needs of the critically injured. Therefore, the designation of one hospital allows that hospital to expend its resources for such necessities as CAT scans, nuclear medicine, arteriography, the necessary intensive care space, as well as the personnel present at all times. It is simply too expensive for every hospital in the community to provide this type of response.

As our system continued to develop and mature, there was a gradual shift, as mentioned, of surgeons toward the regional trauma center if they were interested in this type of surgery.

It was also obvious that for this system to continue to serve the needs of the emergency patients other components mandated by the federal government were essential and uniform access, i.e., "911" was implemented, central dispatch of emergency vehicles was instituted, as well as transfer agreements between institutions transferring patients and our receiving institution.

About the time we thought we had all of these problems solved and the system was functioning smoothly, we then started our MICU program. This is an entirely different situation because everyone feels that he can handle a cardiac patient or ventricular fibrillation. So once again we had another territorial disagreement. How do we solve this problem since we had three hospitals and each of them felt it could handle the cardiac patient? A very unique and interesting solution to this problem occurred.

In Peoria at that time we had two ambulance companies. One of these companies began operating in 1940, and because St. Francis Hospital had the most active ER the majority of patients that the ambulance service cared for over a 30-year period came to St. Francis Hospital. In effect, our institution was essentially supporting that ambulance company. The MICU program now appeared in the community and St. Francis Hospital was named as the resource hospital because at that particular time we had the only board-certified cardiologists on our staff. Methodist Hospital, on the other hand, had just built a new coronary care unit and they were most anxious to utilize this facility. To attempt to counteract the anticipated increased flow of patients of cardiac nature to St. Francis Hospital they purchased the ambulance company that St. Francis Hospital had supported for many years.

There was another ambulance company in our community at that time which was not an extremely well-staffed or well-organized operation. Our hospital felt that we must have adequate ambulance coverage and purchased this company, but this obviously left the third hospital in our community without an ambulance company of their own. The administrators of the three hospitals then met and discussed the situation. These discussions resulted in appointing a board of directors with equal representation from all three hospitals, forming a not-for-profit corporation of these three hospitals and creating a single ambulance company with equal representation and control by all three hospitals. This has brought about some amazing changes in the ambulance delivery in our community, not only from the standpoint of patient care, but also from the improvement of hospital relationships.

As for the cardiac patient, the same type of corporate body solution to the problem was achieved. An advisory board for the MICU program was formed with equal representation from all three hospitals, but since St. Francis Hospital had been designated as the resource hospital, the responsibility for patient care and training of paramedic personnel rested with our institution.

How did categorization affect our paramedic program? In such the same way, that is, the paramedic program in our community is based at all three hospitals. Once our paramedics are certified and working they not only rotate through the three shifts but also through the three hospital ERs so that their experience is not particularly oriented to one group of physicians and nurses, but rather to the community medical resources as a whole. When the paramedics are not on a specific run, they perform their duties in the ERs of each of the three hospitals which enables them to maintain their skills. Not only is this helpful to the paramedics, but it provides additional assistance in the three hospital ERs. A portion of their pay is paid by the hospitals since they are receiving services from these individuals working in the ER.

Has this affected the patient flow in our community? The fears that everyone had never materialized. That is a fact because the patient still has the right of choice of institution. When one keeps this basic American principle in mind, categorization need not interfere with physicians, desires or patient rights. However, a gradual evolution of the delivery of medical services occurs, providing a more efficient and cost-effective solution to this aspect of health services delivery.

Another interesting aspect of categorization has occurred in the community. Approximately 85% of all cancer patients in Peoria are operated upon at St. Francis Hospital. We do not have radiation therapy at our institution. In fact, we do not even have an oncologist at St. Francis Hospital. We do have in our community as excellent a radiation center in Peoria as one will find in the Midwest. This is located at Methodist Hospital. While St. Francis Hospital has adapted its services and equipment to the needs of the emergency patient, Methodist Hospital, on the other hand, has developed its oncology program for the treatment of cancer patients. For example, if a patient requires radiation therapy, it is as simple to accomplish as writing the order "radiation consultation" on the patient's chart. The radiotherapist and the oncologist from Methodist make rounds at the other two institutions every day and there is a very close working relationship between the institutions. As one can see, some rather interesting things have occurred as a result of categorization. We have noticed because of our trauma load that we may not have any available beds in our institution at a given time. On the other hand, patients requiring radiation therapy are occupying beds that could be occupied by our trauma patients and occasionally patients are found in "hall beds" in our institution. When this occurs it is not unusual for the radiotherapist to suggest that the patient be transferred to Methodist Hospital for therapy. There is no objection to this and it obviously frees beds for the trauma patients. The community again benefits from this working relationship between institutions.

The fear still persists, however, that hospitals will be losing patients and money if all of the injured patients are transferred to another institution. Our statistics show that 80% of all patients injured can be treated in the facility in which they are first seen provided there is a system such as exists in Illinois. Only 15% of the patients would have to be transferred to an intermediate category, and only 5% of all of the injured patients are injured severely enough to be transferred to a regional center.

The system in Illinois provides three levels of hospital response capabilities. These are known as (1) local trauma centers where primarily stabilization and resuscitation are carried out for the seriously injured patients who are then transferred. The majority of the injured patients can be treated at this institution and remain there. Approximately 15% of the patients require a level of care higher than that available in the local trauma centers and they are transferred to (2) areawide trauma centers. The third category is the regional trauma center. Approximately 5% of all injured patients in our region are serious enough to require transfer to the regional center. From a practical standpoint if only 5% of the patients have to be transferred to a regional center, and in our region we have 23 hospitals, 80% of the patients are treated at those 23 hospitals. Obviously if only 5% have to be transferred, the effect on the bed census of the local hospitals has been negligible.

A rather interesting development has occurred following categorization in our region. A large percentage of the efforts to organize and implement the categorization process was done on a voluntary basis by the physicians in private practice who identified the need to implement this cost-effective system. In addition to the physicians there is needed at least one hospital administrator and probably the administrator of the regional center to actively implement many of the physicians' decisions regarding this systems approach. That particular hospital administrator must be totally supportive of such things as buying a new x-ray machine, enlarging the ER or dealing with the H.S.A.'s if it is felt additional equipment or building expansion is necessary.

It is of interest to note how a categorization process affects the distribution of patients as a result of a major disaster when a community has more than one hospital. A recent series of incidents in Peoria, Illinois, indicates the effectiveness of proper patient triage and treatment when categorization has been accomplished.

I was recently returning home in my car when I monitored the dispatch of the paramedic units to a location 17 miles outside Peoria. A group of 36 young adults were on a hayrack ride when the tractor and the hayrack went over a 30-foot sheer dropoff. By means of our sophisticated communications system at the regional center we were able to determine the seriousness of the injuries of these 36 people, notify each of the three hospitals of the accident and the type of patients they would be receiving. The most serious and multiply injured patients were sent to St. Francis Hospital, the regional center. The less serious, the simple fractures and lacerations, were sent to one of the other two institutions in Peoria which had been alerted. Shortly after this incident another hayrack accident occurred with 32 people on board. This hayrack was struck broadside by a truck and the same plan was put into effect. When the last person was extricated from beneath the three-ton tractor I returned to St. Francis Hospital expecting to find our ER in a state of utter confusion. I was much surprised, however, to learn that all the patients had been seen, either treated and released, admitted to our ICU for observation, or all diagnostic procedures had been completed and several were in surgery. I do not think that this effective, efficient treatment of over 60 people in a one-hour period involved in a major accident could have occurred without the process of categorization having been implemented.

Categorization has also effected some surprising results in reduction of mortality. Prior to the implementation of this system in 1971 the number of deaths per 1,000 life-threatening accidents in Region 1-B in Illinois was 93. In 1978 the death rate per 1,000 life-threatening accidents had dropped to an amazing 50. This again is the result of the multiple components mandated by the federal government which, when placed on an operational status, can decrease the death rate in serious accident cases.

I was recently asked a question regarding the statistics that we collect in Region 1-B and I think it is essential that I comment upon this aspect of our program. The privacy act has made it extremely difficult for us to gather data. Our situation in Region 1-B in Illinois was one of complete frustration in obtaining the Department of Transportation's statistics regarding highway accidents and injuries. Because of the concern over the privacy act the legal department of the Illinois Department of Transportation felt that they could not release this information to us.

We then were forced to contact the Illinois State Police and manually trace from 1971 through 1978 the microfilm records to pick out our tracer group which was the Class A injuries for the month of June during those years. After obtaining from the Illinois State Police the information, which consisted of the name and the county in which the injuries occurred, it was then necessary to go to each hospital to trace individually those patient records to determine the outcome of their treatment.

We recently had another problem arise in Illinois and it has some reflection upon what Dr. Boyd has requested as the "lead agencies" in the state. Dr. Boyd has felt that the Department of Public Health should be the lead agency; however, the present Director of the Department of Public Health of Illinois has absolutely no interest and has assigned absolutely no priority rating to EMS. Rather, funds have been diverted from EMS to areas which the Director and Associate Director felt were of greater importance. My point is very simply this: Do not allow federal dollars to come to your state and expect them to be utilized to your satisfaction without your input, concern and involvement in the state Department of Public Health.

Self-Evaluation Quiz

1. Oscar Hampton of the American College of Surgeons is considered the pioneer of the approach to the trauma problem.
   a) True
   b) False
2. According to the American College of Surgeons, the optimum response hospital must have 12-hour inhouse surgical specialties and subspecialties.
   a) True
   b) False
3. According to Dr. Boyd, the Department of Public Health should be the lead agency in a state.
   a) True
   b) False
4. It is not necessary to establish transfer agreements before referring patients between hospitals and physicians.
   a) True
   b) False
5. Patient flow in Region 1-B was markedly disrupted by the EMS system.
   a) True
   b) False

Answers on page 289.

Perspective on Pre-Hospital Care for Trauma Patients

Frank Lewis, Jr., M.D.

Objectives

1. To illustrate the problems involved in treating the trauma patient en route to the hospital.
2. To emphasize that the EMT is not the diagnostician and often lives may be saved if the patient is transported immediately.
3. To recognize airway obstruction and intubation techniques and that there be no delay in transport for intravenous placement or other diagnostic and therapeutic regimens.

Although the position I shall state here may be a little bit stronger than that which I actually support, I do think that there are several points in this position that need to be examined closely. The point that I would really like to address is that pre-hospital EMT care does not contribute to survival in trauma. One must have an open mind about this question and be willing to consider your results. Just to illustrate the value of keeping an open mind and taking a fresh look at things, I would cite two instances which illustrate this particular problem.

First is the question of coronary care units in hospitals. Who would ever dream of questioning coronary care units? Who would ever say they do not do any good? Everybody knows that they have intensive nursing and intensive monitoring and everything one could ask for in caring for myocardial infarction patients. Therefore, how could one possibly contend that nursing care in a coronary care unit is not beneficial and does

---

Frank Lewis, Jr., M.D., Associate Professor of Surgery; Surgical Director, Intensive Care Unit, San Francisco General Hospital, Calif.; Founding Member, American Trauma Society.

not save lives? The answer is that it has been done and it is true. For a selected subgroup of patients who have had myocardial infarction, those who do not have significant arrhythmias in the immediate postinfarction period, it appears that patients do at least as well and possibly better if left at home rather than admitted to a hospital coronary care unit. I would gather that this is contrary to what many have been taught and what many think. But there have been some recent studies that seem to show that.

The second instance concerns emergency ambulances — the idea that ambulances should always be given priority to get from any scene of an accident to the nearest hospital in the fastest possible time and should, therefore, be given permission by the law enforcement authorities to break the normal traffic laws in order to do so. That would include going through red lights and through intersections in order to get where they are going. Little Rock, Arkansas, takes the contrary view. In fact, they have adopted the position that ambulances are not emergency vehicles and they cannot break the traffic laws. They cannot go through red lights. They cannot go through intersections marked with stop signs without first stopping, when transporting patients. It is believed that the lives saved by preventing accidents involving ambulances well justify that position. I am sure most of you would not agree with that. But there are contrary points of view which must be considered; in order to decide what is right and what is wrong, you really need to consider your results.

In regard to trauma care, I think the fundamental question underlying this whole area is to ask: From what cause do trauma patients die? If you hope to make inroads in this with pre-hospital or in-hospital care, you should ask yourself, what is it you are trying to treat? What do you want the EMTs to be trained to do? Because if the patient is going to do just as well either way, then the expense of having an EMT training program and of having expensive monitoring equipment and communications is really not worthwhile. Basically, we are all in a business which is more and more costly. The government or the insurance companies or the public is going to demand of us that we make it less expensive or at least prevent the costs from escalating so rapidly and that we justify what we are doing as being cost-effective.

In trauma patients, statistics from numerous centers over the years have shown the same thing. For most traumatized patients, the greatest single cause of death will be from head injury. Approximately one half of all trauma deaths will be the result of head injury. Very little progress has been made in that area over the last 50 years. Most of the treatment for head injury is supportive treatment. There are very few specific procedures that can be done to salvage a patient with head injury. He either has an injury which is too severe and it will kill him or he has an injury which is less severe and if you support him long enough he will survive. If he has a space-occupying traumatic lesion, it can be drained neurosurgically. But by and large the mortality from head injuries has not changed in 50 years. Edema following trauma is the major cause of death in patients who do not have massive tissue destruction right away. But that is not something that occurs within the first few hours. So the role of the EMT in doing anything to influence it is fairly minimal. Thus, pre-hospital care for head injury will not be beneficial except in so far as the head injury causes other problems for which you can support the patient. In particular, if it causes loss of control of airway, loss of respiratory effort, and you can support the patient by intubating and breathing for him, then you can do something. But for the head injury itself, nothing can be done in the ambulance. Of the remaining patients, if you look at the cause of death and consider what kills patients in the immediate peri-injury period, either from the time of pickup to the hospital or in the first 24 hours in the hospital, the answer is really twofold: either bleeding or immediate airway problems of one sort or another.

Bleeding typically is from internal injuries, either in the chest or more commonly in the abdomen. Airway problems occur either because the patient asphyxiates because he cannot maintain an open airway or because he aspirates massively because his airway was not protected and because of his head injury or a fracture in the maxillofacial area, he could not control his airway and prevent aspiration when he vomited. Of all patients who reach the hospital, the chance of dying from hemorrhage is quite low. Although this represents the second most common cause of death in the peri-hospital period, once the patient gets to a competent hospital where emergency services are available, less than 5% of all deaths result from bleeding.

So we immediately have a contrast. Death from bleeding is a frequent cause of pre-hospital mortality, but is an infrequent cause of in-hospital mortality. This is not particularly surprising since very little can be done in an ambulance to control bleeding when it is coming from an internal source. Obviously, you can control bleeding from an extremity or from a fracture site. But when you consider that most of the patients who die from bleeding die before they get to the hospital, I think you must then examine the question of time of transit.

What can be done about that particular problem? There are really only three things possible. First, get the patient to the hospital quickly, so that you have someone there with the necessary facilities to back you up and take care of the patient. Second, start an intravenous drip and give the patient fluids en route to the hospital. As many of you know, that is easier said than done. Trying to start intravenous fluids in an ambulance which is bouncing along a road is difficult. Starting intravenous fluids in any patient who is hypovolemic is difficult because he is vasoconstricted and it is difficult to find his veins. If the patient is bleeding, and if he is going to die of a bleeding injury, it would be my contention that you would be better off not to waste time trying to get an IV started at the scene and delaying your pick-up and transfer of the patient but, rather, to get the patient to the hospital as quickly as possible so that definitive care can be given. It is my personal feeling that starting IVs in a traumatized patient and trying to give him fluids is counter-productive. The time expended, if you are delaying transfer, is really not worthwhile. It is preferable to get the patient to the hospital where something can be done for him that you cannot do. You cannot open the abdomen, you cannot get at the source of the bleeding. The third possibility is use of the Medical Anti-Shock Trouser, or MAST suit. We in San Francisco do not use it, because San Francisco is basically a small town, 7 miles square. The hospital is slightly to the east of center but relatively centrally located and everything is brought to one place. As a result, the average time for an ambulance run is six to seven minutes. It would take longer to get the MAST suit unzipped and on the patient than it would to get the patient to the hospital where he can receive definitive care. In a rural setting, where one has longer ambulance runs and is dealing with patients who are hypovolemic from abdominal trauma or extremity trauma, probably the MAST suit does have a role. Again, there has been very little evidence shown that, in fact, it can be used effectively. But at least on a theoretical basis, it would appear that it may have something to offer. As with everything, there is a trade-off. Clearly, when you have a patient who has some degree of respiratory compromise, you cannot use the MAST suit with the abdominal part of it zipped up and inflated because, if you do, you will compromise ventilation and the patient will be worse than he was before from a respiratory point of view. You must recognize that if you choose to use the MAST suit, the patient must have either fairly normal respiratory function, or you must be willing to intubate and ventilate him with positive pressure during the course of transit. So, the MAST suit has a place. It does one thing fairly well, that is, gives the patient in effect an autotransfusion and helps eliminate bleeding, but it compromises respiratory function. I think in certain situations it may well be useful. But when it takes longer to put it on than it does to get the patient to the hospital, then I think it does not have a role.

The other cause of death is airway problems. If you look at all of the things that are available, by and large, most of them are worth very little. The one definitive action in protecting the airway is inserting an endotracheal tube. Inserting nasal and oral airways is in many cases going to make the patient vomit and increase the chance of aspiration. Someone who is skilled in maintaining an airway can do more with their hands, positioning the head and the chin, than any nasal or oral airway can possibly accomplish. If you really want to protect the patient and give him positive pressure ventilation, you need an endotracheal tube to do it. To me, that is the one thing that really could make a difference in pre-hospital care because that is the other major cause of death in trauma patients, airway problems. So if you are asking what do EMTs do and how can they be trained to really affect mortality in trauma patients, my answer would be to forget all the impractical theory and teach them how to insert endotracheal tubes in a patient who is unconscious or who has a compromised airway, because that represents a very specific skill which would have real value in lowering mortality. We find that among trauma victims who come in unconscious, the frequency of aspiration is approximately 15% to 20% and mortality from aspiration is about one third. No matter what you do, if you have aspirated gastric contents, it is a bad lesion. It is imperative to prevent it before it occurs, and you can do that only by having an endotracheal tube with an airtight seal in the patient.

The next consideration is where the patient should be taken. This is not directly EMT care, but it is the question that all of you need to consider. The biggest problem we have in this country today is recognizing that all hospitals are not equivalent in their ability to treat traumatized patients. A major study authored by John West is about to be published, in which he examined the mortality from trauma in a group of patients in Orange County, California. He found that between 20% and 25% of those patients died needlessly of injuries as simple as a ruptured spleen that were totally preventable and bleeding complications that were not recognized and treated properly.

That is not something that you can do anything about directly, but you can influence it by recognizing that hospitals are different. In your own particular area you should select a hospital for traumatized patients which has full emergency capability. You should work within your area to develop regional plans for hospitals that will have trauma capability, so that when patients are brought in, they will not lie around for hours, waiting for a surgeon, an operating room team or someone who can diagnose the problem and deal with it effectively. To me, that is the second part of the equation, when you start discussing whether EMT care is useful: what kind of hospital do you have to back you up? Where are you going to take the patient who is a trauma victim once you have picked him up?

Trying to teach EMTs to diagnose or to treat in the ambulance is counterproductive. It is often difficult for us to determine what is wrong with a patient once he gets to the emergency room, where we have all of the diagnostic adjuncts available. I think much of the time and training that goes into teaching EMTs to be diagnosticians is a waste of time. You should look at the things you can really do which will prevent mortality and the things you can be trained to do skillfully, and that is what you should do. Obviously, no one is going to argue with the simple, quick treatment such as putting on pressure dressings to control bleeding, splinting fractures in carrying patients, looking out for cervical spine fractures and, if it is easy, starting an IV. Most of you, however, would not be comfortable giving fluids in the volumes that are required to really treat hypovolemic shock. If someone is bleeding rapidly, you are going to have to give him 2 to 3 liters in one-half hour. Most of you would not be comfortable doing that because you are not accustomed to doing it. You have no way of monitoring the patient during the process. If you have made the wrong diagnosis, you might make it worse by that sort of fluid administration.

The administration of drugs intravenously is virtually worthless in the trauma victim. So having an IV available to give drugs is really counterproductive. You probably create more problems than you treat. In the cardiac patient, that may be different. I do not deal with that. But in the trauma victim, the name of the game is replacement of intravascular volume and, if you are going to treat the patient effectively, control of the bleeding and provision of definitive therapy.

Cardiopulmonary resuscitation in the hypovolemic patient is ineffective. Closed chest CPR does no good in the exsanguinated patient because if the heart is empty, there is nothing to compress between the sternum and the spine. CPR is effective in cardiogenic problems because those patients have high venous filling pressures, they have normal or increased intravascular volumes, and the heart fills very readily. It tends to be dilated and overdistended, so that when you administer closed chest CPR, you have a distended myocardium that you can compress between the sternum and the spine and CPR is very effective. But when the patient is exsanguinated and the heart is empty, pushing on the sternum does no good whatsoever. The only thing you can do which has any effect is open chest CPR and that is only marginally effective until you get volume into the patient. You cannot resuscitate someone who has arrested from hemorrhagic shock. They must get volume in and they must get it in rapidly. It would be my contention that you would be far better off to get patients to a hospital, where they can open the chest, administer massage, put in cutdowns with large-bore lines and get that volume into the patient. We have just recently reviewed our past five years of experience at San Francisco General Hospital, looking at the results of resuscitation in patients who arrive dead on arrival by all parameters. These were patients who were arrested, not breathing, when they came into the emergency room. There were 173 of them over a five-year period. The ultimate salvage rate in these patients was 19%. That is not great but it is better than zero. One cannot do that in an ambulance. One must get the patient to a trauma center or to a hospital where people are available who can do all of the more complicated things that cannot be done in an ambulance. If you waste time getting the patient to the hospital, you are only going to prevent the possibility of later resuscitation because he will have an irreversible heart and brain injury.

The other part of pre-hospital trauma care is to establish a good airway, prevent aspiration and ventilate the patient effectively. In my mind, the most important element in EMT training is to teach EMTs to recognize airway problems, to intubate when it is required for the protection of the unconscious patient and to ventilate patients effectively in transit to the hospital. Beyond that, I think much of the training effort and the time that goes into it serves only to increase the expense of medical care without really improving the results.

I think all of you should question just what are the results we are generating as a result of large-scale EMT training programs. What are we doing for the patient? For example, we could talk about the use of monitors in the ambulance for the trauma victim. I think this also has very little value. A hand on the femoral pulse is more important, because whether or not there is an EKG rhythm, if the patient is not perfusing, you should be instituting cardiac massage. If the patient has an effective pulse, it does not really matter what the rhythm is, you do not need to treat it on the way in.

What makes a difference? How can we affect survival? What kills patients? What can we be trained to do competently and efficiently to really help the trauma victim? These are the vital questions that must be considered.

I think there are two arguments that strongly point to the need for trauma centers and for regionalization of trauma care. The first is that trauma affects young people much more than it affects old people. Three fourths of trauma patients are under 40 years of age; whereas virtually all cancer, heart disease, stroke patients are over 50 years of age. So in terms of the years of productive life left to them, trauma has far more impact than any of those other diseases which have received far greater government support in research and implementation funding than trauma does. That is one of the real tragedies, I think, of the federal policy with regard to health care.

Second, in terms of absolute mortality, the primary cause of death in patients under 45 years of age is trauma. For that reason, that is where we should be putting our attention. There is no doubt in my mind that if the numbers were gathered and were available, and if one has effective trauma centers, then one could show effective salvage of patients in that productive age group and in the great majority of those patients the return to the same level of function as they had prior to the traumatic injury. If you examine the recent paper by Dr. West, showing that in Orange County, California, for every 100 patients dying, 22 or 23 of them had totally preventable death had they been taken to a competently equipped hospital when they were first injured, and you extrapolate those numbers nationwide, with 50,000 deaths from automobile accidents, the numbers are staggering. When you see that one fifth of those patients could have been saved by appropriate regional trauma care, including the paramedic system and the hospital base, that is a phenomenal number. That clearly would be a cost-effective number because the 20% you would be saving are people who are young and are productive, and they could get back to the same level of function they had before. Having a ruptured spleen and having it taken out usually entails a hospital stay of five to six days. After a one- to two-month convalescence, the patient returns to normal function. Having a lacerated liver is the same. Most of the problems you treat that cause mortality are not disabling injuries for the rest of the patient's life. They are not things that affect the patient's function. There certainly are cord injuries and other injuries that are permanent. But the great majority of traumatic injuries that kill people are crisis situations which, once treated, do not result in permanent disability. The amount of nonproductive political hassling that has gone on over the last ten years in this question is inexcusable. Basically we are hung up on political jurisdictions and economic questions. There is no doubt about the way to go, in terms of medical care. But we are hung up because no one wants to be called the nontrauma hospital. Everyone wants to have the trauma business. The administrators all want to have an emergency room but none of them want to put the money into it to make it a comprehensive emergency room. It is time that the political establishment recognizes where the real problem is and starts to address it. This question of pre-hospital care is part of all of that.

Self-Evaluation Quiz

1. The greatest single cause of death in most traumatized patients is:
   a) Renal contusion
   b) Myocardial rupture
   c) Head injury
   d) Rupture of liver
2. In considering a patient with acute trauma the following is true:
   a) In patients who reach the hospital there is a less than 5% chance of dying from hemorrhage
   b) Bleeding is frequently from internal injuries
   c) In patients with major maxillofacial fractures intubation to prevent aspiration may be necessary
   d) All of the above
3. Inserting nasal and oral airways in many patients with head injury may induce vomiting and increase chances of inspiration.
   a) True
   b) False
4. In a large city an ambulance driver confronted with a patient in shock should:
   a) Delay transfer to the hospital until an intravenous line is started
   b) Open the abdomen or chest to tie off the bleeders

   c) Transport the patient immediately and attempt IV line for rapid fluid replacement en route
   d) Place the MAST suit, especially in patients with decompensated respiratory function
5. Endotracheal intubation is a life-saving technique that will decrease pre-hospital mortality if performed by skilled EMTs.
   a) True
   b) False
6. Trauma is the primary cause of death in patients under 45 years. This makes it important to:
   a) Provide more funds for excellent trauma centers
   b) Provide more staff and good surgical backup
   c) Regionalize trauma centers according to demographic studies
   d) All of the above
7. It has recently been reported that 20% of patients die needlessly from preventable complications of trauma.
   a) True
   b) False

Answers on page 289.

Debate

Resolved: Pre-Hospital Decompression of Tension Pneumothorax Is Desirable

Affirmative: Norman E. McSwain, Jr., M.D.
Negative: Kenneth L. Mattox, M.D.

Affirmative

There is no question that a pneumothorax and, in particular, a tension pneumothorax, is treated by reduction of the intrathoracic pressure. This can be accomplished either by gaining access to the pleural space through the second intercostal space at the midclavicular line by inserting a small tube or a needle or by accessing it through the sixth, seventh or eighth intercostal space by a large-bore chest tube. The latter is much more applicable when in the emergency department and when treating a hemothorax. The former is much more applicable when in the field or when treating an isolated pneumothorax because the smaller diameter of the small-bore chest tube or the small needle will obviously not remove blood and clots that occur with the hemothorax. Also, it is difficult to manage the larger tube in the field because it is cumbersome and requires surgical instruments.

The question has arisen in the past and is the subject of this debate: should tension pneumothorax be treated in the prehospital phase of emergency medical care or should it be reserved for the emergency department and the skill of the

---

Norman E. McSwain, Jr., M.D.,* Associate Professor of Surgery, Tulane University School of Medicine, New Orleans, La. and Kenneth L. Mattox, M.D.,* Associate Professor of Surgery, Baylor College of Medicine, Houston, Tex.; Deputy Chief of Surgery and Director of Emergency Surgical Services, Ben Taub General Hospital, Houston.

*Member, Board of Directors, American Trauma Society.

surgeon? Since the mode of treatment is so well accepted, what are the reasons for it not being used in the field?

Several have been proposed. The time required for transport of the patient to the hospital is only five to ten minutes; therefore, such a procedure can easily be delayed for that period of time. This is fallacious for the following reasons:

1. A tension pneumothorax produces relatively rapid anoxia. Brain death occurs within four to six minutes after onset of any type of anoxia.

2. Five- to ten-minute transport time. Yes, five to ten minutes may be possible if one is close to the hospital, but that is from the time the wheels start to roll until the time the wheels come to a stop in front of the hospital. That does not count (a) evaluation time prior to extrication, (b) extrication time, (c) loading the patient in the ambulance, (d) starting the appropriate IV fluids and utilization of other therapies, such as pneumatic trousers, or (e) off-loading the patient after arrival at the hospital and rolling the patient to the emergency room.

Taking all these factors into consideration, you are not five to ten minutes away from the hospital. You are really 20 to 45 minutes away. This is true only if the patient is transported to the closest available hospital. Categorization is the name of the game. The patient is transported to the closest *appropriate* hospital, which is probably more than five to ten minutes away. For those of you working in rural areas, you may be transporting the patient not 5 to 10 minutes but much longer than that, possibly as long as 30 to 45 minutes from the time the wheels start to roll until the time the wheels come to a stop at the hospital.

Another reason frequently offered for not using a chest tube or some other type of pneumothorax device in the field is that the diagnosis of a tension pneumothorax is difficult and requires an x-ray. Dr. Mattox reported in the February 1978 issue of *Emergency Product News* that he reviewed paramedic runs in which over 90% of the cases were overdiagnosed, that were just a simple pneumothorax. I submit that this is a question not of the procedure but of inappropriate training of the personnel. If one uses the proper parameters for diagnosing a tension pneumothorax, that is, (1) unilateral absent breath sounds, (2) deviation of the trachea away from the absent breath sounds, (3) distended neck veins, (4) cyanosis and possibly subcutaneous emphysema, an EMT-P in the field will make the appropriate diagnosis. But let us say that he does not. Let us say that it is only a pneumothorax and not a tension pneumothorax. What is the treatment for a pneumothorax? It is still decompression.

The issue here is not to spend considerable time in the field delaying transportation of the patient to the hospital, but rather to stabilize the patient adequately and, if appropriate, then to decompress the compromised lung. There is certainly a significant amount of skill and training required in the diagnosis of arrhythmias and the treatment of cardiac patients, utilization of drugs in treating their cardiac condition, reading electrocardiograms and other advanced pre-hospital care. If an EMT-P can be trained to utilize these skills in the treatment of cardiac care, including injection of anticardiac medications, why can we not teach him to diagnose and treat a tension pneumothorax in the field?

Another problem that has been raised is skill deterioration. There are those who say that skill deterioration is such that when the time comes for utilization of learned skills, the trained EMT-P will not be able to accomplish it properly because the procedure was used so rarely. Every aspect of a paramedic's skills and knowledge is subject to rapid deterioration if not utilized and if he does not keep abreast of the latest information and refresh his knowledge periodically. The relief of a tension pneumothorax is no exception. Just as an individual trained in cardiopulmonary resuscitation and defibrillation must review those techniques periodically, so must an individual trained in the diagnosis and treatment of a pneumothorax also review these skills and knowledge periodically.

In 1971, when I was working at an automobile race track, a TR-6 automobile crashed into a wooden retaining wall. The car was impacted on the driver's side and this produced a pneumothorax. Evaluation and stabilization at the trackside hospital, which is not unlike roadside evaluation and stabilization of a patient, was accomplished. The patient's shock was treated with intravenous Ringer's lactate. At that time, we were unaware of the benefits of the MAST ® suit, at least I was. A pneumothorax was found to be present and a tension rapidly

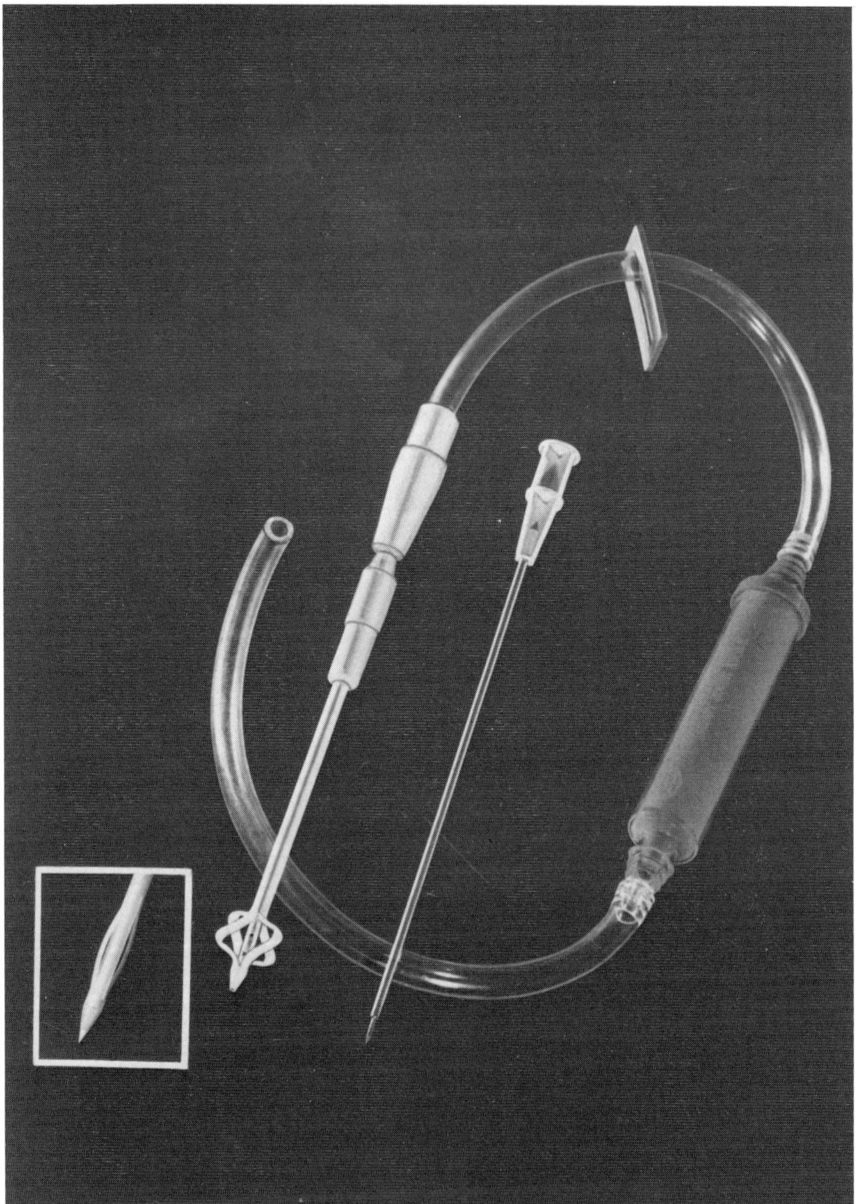

FIGURE 1.

developed. The small needle which I inserted in the second intercostal space midclavicular line was not enough to evacuate and relieve the problem of the tension.

Following partial stabilization was a high speed ride to the hospital. I was frustrated and afraid because I knew what was wrong with the patient and I knew that I did not have the equipment to treat it appropriately. I feared the patient was going to die and I could not do anything about it. I was afraid because of the high speed ambulance ride. I decided at that time that I would try to devise some method to treat this situation which would benefit me the next time I was in that situation and which would also avoid the high speed ambulance ride and the frustration of not being able to handle the patient but, more importantly, to help those of you who are seeing it much more frequently to manage this type of patient. The McSwain Dart ® was the result (Figs. 1 and 2).

Should paramedics utilize invasive mechanisms to relieve a tension pneumothorax? Yes, they should. To deprive a patient

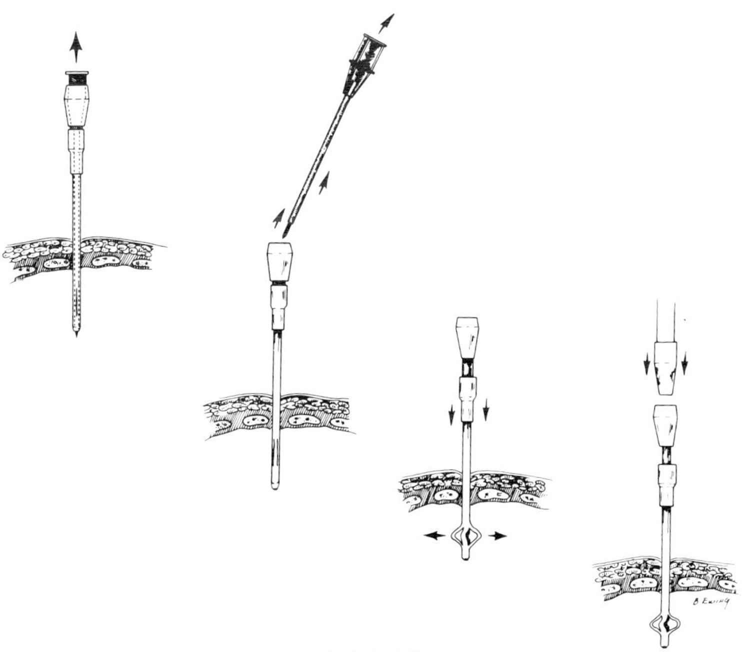

FIGURE 2.

of a life-saving treatment when a competent paramedic can be trained effectively to accomplish some relief is to stop the progress of EMS in the United States and to deprive our patients of needed pre-hospital care.

Negative

Trauma care, and emergency medical services (EMS) in particular, has suffered from emotionalism, gadgetry, saturation marketing, proprietorship, entrepreneurism, overzealous sales, bandwagon tactics, "me-tooism" and "I also-ranism." Especially in the pre-hospital phase, EMS techniques and device utilization have very little supporting scientific data as to efficacy. Fortunately, the Medical Device Act of 1976 began to protect the consumer and the physician from fraudulent advertising and unsafe medical devices. However, the Food and Drug Administration's device section is required to clear medical devices appearing on the market only after January 1978. For a device or instrument to be placed on the market, the following questions should be asked: Is there a need? What is the harm:benefit ratio? Are there potential hazards? Are there known or reported complications? Is there efficacy? Does this particular device fill the proposed need? Is there utility? Can everyone use this device with equal facility, skill and safety?

Several questions arise, specifically as they relate to the pre-hospital decompression of a tension pneumothorax. First, in civilian EMS, do people die (especially pre-hospital) or suffer temporary or permanent morbidity from tension pneumothorax or undrained pneumothorax or a straightforward hemopneumothorax? Second, in civilian EMS, can the skills to diagnose tension pneumothorax accurately and reproducibly be taught to a paramedic, a mobile intensive care unit nurse, an emergency room physician or even a traumatologist? Third, in civilian EMS, what are the medicolegal responsibilities for performing a necessary invasive maneuver incorrectly or causing some injury? When that invasive maneuver is performed but was not indicated, is there liability? Fourth, in the trauma patient does the time it takes in the field to insert and secure a needle in the chest justify its use?

As far as indications are concerned, in analyzing medical examiners' data with regard to victims of automobile accidents, gunshot wounds or even spontaneous pneumothorax, a patient in the morgue who had tension pneumothorax and was dead on arrival at the hospital is rarely, if ever, reported. People very rarely die (especially pre-hospital) of known tension pneumothorax.

What are the physics of a tension pneumothorax? The normal atmospheric pressure is approximately 14 pounds per square inch (psi) at sea level. In the patient who develops a tension pneumothorax, either spontaneously or secondary to penetration or a rupture from barotrauma, considerable pressure in the pleural space is required to deviate the mediastinum and cause cardiac arrest. Only when there is endotracheal intubation or mask ventilation with the further creation of a valve mechanism is the mediastinum deviated. In the old days of the Drinker® Tank during the polio era, many patients had tension pneumothoraces that would go untreated for days and the patient would have little evidence of cardiac compromise. So, only in that patient who has an endotracheal airway inserted with its accompanying forced positive ventilation do tension pneumothoraces become serious threats.

Concerning the atmospheric pressure, several questions arise: First, what pressure in psi is required on the mediastinum (as supported by the literature) to move the mediastinum enough to critically kink the vena cava as the mediastinum is "pushed" to the other side? Second, what psi has been measured in experiments and in observed clinical tension pneumothorax? Third, what are the tolerable limits of positive psi in the pleural space? Fourth, what is the normal, negative or positive psi recorded in the normal, the pneumothorax and the tension pneumothorax pleural space?

As it relates to safety, one must ask the question: Are there particular conditions which simulate a pneumothorax or tension pneumothorax? Yes, there are. These include spontaneous pneumothorax, cavitary pulmonary tuberculosis, advanced pulmonary emphysema, pulmonary blebs, giant pulmonary bullae and a bronchopleural fistula with loculated empyema.

In a review of eight centers which I visited, the percent of physician misdiagnoses of tension pneumothorax approaches 85%, that is, the physicians (who may be the ones training the paramedic) frequently misdiagnose a straightforward pneumothorax as a tension pneumothorax.

If we look at the device itself, we are inserting a small trochar into the pleural space. We must recall that 15% to 20% of the population already have pleural symphysis. Without diagnostic confirmation of a pneumothorax, the blind insertion of an instrument into this space results in problems. Because the location of the tip of the trochar is unknown, perforation of the lung, diaphragm, inferior vena cava, heart, aorta, trachea, liver, spleen, stomach or colon may occur when the "shish-kabab" trochar chest tubes (or any variant thereof) are inserted blindly. Ironically, trained and experienced thoracic surgeons and traumatologists are the most vocal in asking for the nonuse and even the recall of these trochar chest tubes. In a survey conducted in south Texas, such trochar chest tubes were advocated mainly by those with very little experience in pleural or thoracic physiology who only occasionally or rarely inserted a chest tube. There are problems encountered in all emergency rooms with the routine insertion of a tube thoracostomy. Such problems might logically be predicted to occur with the McSwain Dart.

Finally, there are a number of devices and techniques which may be used or can be performed, but which may or may not be indicated. One can give an enema to a patient in the pre-hospital phase, but just because it can be done, should it be done? Of course not!

A number of faddish techniques have become uncommon or result in no clinical improvement. These include such things as internal mammary artery ligation for angina, nephroplexy for ptotic kidneys, copper bracelets for the treatment of arthritis, Lydia Pinkham ® tonic for the treatment of menopausal women, thoracotomy in the emergency center for dead patients, cricothyroidotomy, augmentation mammoplasty, membrane oxygenation for respiratory insufficiency, estrogen therapy and even castration for stage A-1 and B carcinoma of the prostate, gastric freezing for gastrointestinal bleeding and carotid body excision for treatment of asthma. Perhaps a number of our pre-hospital interventions should likewise become obsolete.

In summary, in analyzing the four issues related to the development of a medical device, the available epidemiologic data do not support the need for pre-hospital thoracic decompression. There is no question that the development of a specific instrument for thoracic decompression can be safely used pre hospital and in the emergency center; however, many thoracic surgeons abhor the use of the trochar. A needle, knife, chest tube or the McSwain Dart can indeed decompress a tension pneumothorax if the instrument is placed accurately and the condition diagnosed properly. Still, the best place for thoracic decompression is in the hospital — not in the field.

In answer to the specific four questions as they relate to the pre-hospital use of thoracic decompression, the presently available devices for pre-hospital thoracic decompression are gadgets in search of an indication; they increase the pre-hospital "busy work" and delay adequate and proper therapy.

Rebuttal: Dr. McSwain

Dr. Mattox seems to advocate the "grab them and run to the hospital" technique, so that the invasive skills can be accomplished by a physician. I do not believe that these skills are hallowed and reserved for physicians only, but that they can be carried out in the field under medical control prior to an adequate stabilization and transportation.

The question of whether a pneumothorax or a tension pneumothorax can be diagnosed on autopsy specimens is real. I do not know whether any of you have spent much time in the morgue, but a tension pneumothorax is a clinical diagnosis. When you open the chest, the classical Y-shaped incision to do a postmortem examination, the lung can then either re-expand or it can collapse. The pathologists with whom I have discussed this problem say they cannot diagnose a tension pneumothorax in the autopsy room. Perhaps Dr. Mattox's pathologists can do so.

The question of how many psi is necessary to kink the vena cava I do not think is a real consideration in tension pneumothorax. Several recent publications have questioned if this kinking actually occurs or not and even if it does it does not represent a threat in a tension pneumothorax. So perhaps this is not a problem at all. People are beginning to think that the increased right heart pressure is not due to kinking of the vena cava, but rather to the increased intrapleural pressure.

Dr. Mattox mentioned that 85% of the physicians could not diagnose a tension pneumothorax. I resubmit to you that this is not a procedural problem but a training problem. Just as the criticism of the esophageal obturator airway (EOA) has been made that it is put into the trachea too often, if an EMT-P or an EMT-A cannot recognize when the EOA is placed in the trachea by listening to the chest, he should not have it in his hands anyway. This is not a problem with the device, but rather a problem of training.

Where is the integrity of an EMS system that does not allow a trained individual to perform to the state of the art? There is no question that a tension pneumothorax is a real problem in the field. Certainly, it is rare in the field but when it occurs it is real. I see no reason why we should not train pre-hospital personnel adequately to use these skills. One who advocates less than this, in my estimation, lacks the courage to accept the challenge of advancement.

When faced with a problem in emergency medicine or in any other branch of medicine, we must consider the patient's feelings. A patient in the field who is anoxic, who is anxious, who cannot breathe well because of his hypoxia — we need to be concerned for his humanitarian problems. We cannot ignore these and develop a callous attitude toward them and just say, "Well, that is all right, let us just get him to the hospital and maybe he will get better and maybe he will not die en route." We must have one foot firmly planted in biology and the other in the humanities in order to properly treat and care for our patients.

Rebuttal: Dr. Mattox

During the past two years, we have had the good fortune of having at least eight different national symposia or regional workshops sponsored by the Department of Health, Education and Welfare, Division of Emergency Medical Services. At each of these, there has been a trauma workshop. For those of you who attended the workshops in your own regions, you will recall that during that trauma workshop, virtually every traumatologist in the country who sees any volume of trauma at all supports the contention that in trauma, in opposition to some of the cardiac patients, perhaps the old "grab them and run" philosophy is not bad at all. Indeed, all of us have seen considerable time wasted in the field by paramedics or "pseudosurrogate physicians" who wished to stabilize a patient who could not be stabilized in the field for a variety of reasons. Starting intravenous fluids, yes; maintaining an airway, yes; stopping the flow of hemorrhage, yes. Beyond that it is imperative to transfer the trauma victim to the hospital as quickly as possible.

I would like to thank Dr. McSwain for pointing out that in tension pneumothorax the vena cava may, indeed, not be kinked. Dr. McSwain has stated that those people who die of tension pneumothorax die of decreased cardiac output. I am really not aware of any increased right heart pressure that has been reported with tension pneumothorax.

I have no quarrel with the fact that we do have a training problem with emergency nurses, emergency physicians and with paramedics. However, those are the facts with which we are dealing across the United States today. These not only relate to problems of tension pneumothorax but when to remove MAST trousers, when to remove esophageal obturator airway and the like.

In our objective to provide optimal care during the pre-hospital phase, just what percentage of the gross national product are we willing to spend in performing such tricks simply because they can be done but whose benefits are marginal? In one city consideration (maybe tongue in cheek, but somewhat seriously) is being given to placing a patient on portable cardiopulmonary bypass using a membrane oxygenator and transporting him via helicopter. Another neighboring state is proposing to place a cardiopulmonary bypass in a van that moves halfway across the state for treatment of cardiac failure. I submit that these may not be cost-effective in today's cost-containment-conscious community.

Finally, in those patients with observed tension pneumothorax who have been in our trauma center during the past year, systolic blood pressure of approximately 70 to 80 mm Hg has been observed. This blood pressure is tolerated quite well by all the physiologic adjustments to hypotension. So, I submit to you that in the pre-hospital phase, as Dr. McSwain has correctly pointed out, the "grab them and run" philosophy with stabilization en route, especially for the patient with the tension pneumothorax, has a great deal of merit.

Endotracheal Tube Vs. Esophageal Obturator

Don M. Benson, M.D.

Objectives

1. To list, describe and discuss the three aspects of airway control.
2. To discuss the advantages and disadvantages of the esophageal obturator airway, the esophagogastric tube airway and the endotracheal tube.
3. To provide examples of specific situations where an endotracheal tube is definitely superior.
4. To provide examples of when the esophageal obturator airway or the esophagogastric tube airway is superior.
5. To discuss the relative feasibility of training large numbers of rescue personnel in insertion of the appliances.

Introduction

I shall allude to endotracheal intubation and discuss my thoughts about the feasibility with which it can be accomplished. I would ask you to consider the differences between esophagogastric tube insertion and endotracheal intubation, where one is applicable and where the other would be more optimally applicable.

First, it is necessary to define specifically what we are trying to do when we approach a patient with the goal of controlling his airway. I submit that there are really three components to airway control. In order to find out how the esophagogastric tube airway (EGTA) or the esophageal obturator airway (EOA)

Don M. Benson, M.D., Clinical Associate Professor of Anesthesiology, University of Pittsburgh; Medical Director, Stark County Paramedic Training Program, Canton, Ohio.

and the endotracheal tube (ETT) relate to one another, we must look at how each of them accomplishes the three goals we want to achieve with airway control. The three goals are as follows:

1. Oxygenation. Our primary goal in approaching the patient who is suffering from an airway problem is to oxygenate that patient.
2. Ventilation.
3. Protecting the lungs from soilage by foreign matter, whether it be gastric contents, teeth, steering wheels, cement, gravel or whatever — in other words, protection from pulmonary aspiration.

The second issue to discuss in order to discern how the EGTA and the ETT relate to one another is the relative incidence of complications.

The third and probably the most essential issue is the feasibility of training large numbers of rescue personnel in these various techniques. We can have the best instrument in the world, but if adequate training for the personnel who must use the instruments is not feasible, it is of absolutely no value.

Goals of Airway Control

Oxygenation

In the field situation, the most immediately effective way to improve a patient's oxygenation is to raise the inspired oxygen concentration. It can be done easily with either the EGTA or the ETT. If the ETT is in, put a self-refilling bag-mask unit on it, with an auxiliary oxygen source, and ventilate the patient. The inspired oxygen concentration rises and, hopefully, the patient's arterial oxygen concentration will rise and his oxygen transport will be improved. Likewise, if using an EGTA or an EOA, simply ventilate the patient with an oxygen-rich source. In terms of the first goal, I do not really see much difference between the EGTA and the ETT.

Ventilation

Consider the criteria necessary to accomplish pulmonary ventilation. First, obtain a clear pathway for gas to travel from the ambient atmosphere or the oxygen-rich mixture down to the pulmonary alveoli. If there is a banana or vomitus or other material in the way, remove it — it is imperative to obtain a clear air passageway.

A pressure gradient must be created between the ambient atmosphere and the pulmonary alveoli. The way this is accomplished is to raise the ambient pressure with a self-refilling bag-valve unit or whatever your favorite positive pressure resuscitation device happens to be.

The ETT, if inserted skillfully and swiftly, secures a patent airway between the atmosphere and the trachea. The EGTA does not do that by itself. It must be accompanied by additional maneuvers to raise the tongue from the back of the throat; if there is other foreign matter residing in the pharynx, this must be removed through maneuvers other than simply inserting the appliance. So I submit that in this case the ETT perhaps is superior.

As for creating a pressure gradient with the ETT, if the cuff is inflated, then one has the lungs pretty much at his mercy. One can put 200 lb pressure down there, if one has a device for doing so and if one wants to do it; one has a closed gastight system and can ventilate to one's heart's content and, incidentally, to the patient's detriment if one does not do it properly.

On the other hand, with the EGTA or the EOA, there is an additional problem before one can really raise the pressure gradient — securing a gas-tight fit with the mask on the patient's face. The masks designed for use with these appliances are very well designed. They do not have many of the problems associated with getting a gas tight fit that some of the older, less sophisticated appliances had. Yet, I submit that in less skilled hands, and certainly in more demanding circumstances, such as a shotgun wound of the face, it is difficult to get a good mask fit. In cases such as this, the ETT is probably better.

With regard to ventilation, I would like to raise the issue of compliance (distensibility) of the chest. If the patient has a railroad car lying on top of his chest, it is going to be very difficult to inspire. If the patient is in the middle of a severe asthmatic attack, it is very difficult to inspire. With the ETT one can help overcome some of the compliance difficulties perhaps a little more easily than with the EGTA simply because one has a gas-tight system.

Protection

Finally, regarding protection of the trachea from soilage, the ETT is a superior appliance most of the time, although I have seen occasions where the ventilation device was removed from the ETT, the patient vomited and the vomitus went down the ETT. So it is not 100% effective, but the EGTA does protect the patient from the hazard of regurgitation of gastric contents. I really think it is a godsend in that regard. I feel it is a real breakthrough and I wholeheartedly endorse its use in that respect.

However, another facet we must consider is its failure to protect the trachea from soilage by material coming from above, such as blood from a facial fracture or teeth.

Complications

As one studies the literature, one finds little information on complications. Isolated case reports here and there may be found. One will find a series of data which suggests that the complication rate is small really for both endotracheal intubation and EOA or EGTA use. We all have anecdotal information about complications associated with both. So I submit that on the issue of complications, there is really no point on which to take a position. There is no evidence to support one over the other.

Feasibility

Training in EGTA or in EOA use is not as demanding as training in endotracheal intubation. However, I would also submit to you that training in endotracheal intubation is by no means impossible. Last year we reviewed 45,000 ambulance runs, comprised of 11 ambulance services. These were substantially different services. The smallest service had 38 runs per month and the largest service 1,600 runs monthly. So there is a wide variety of services.

In this population, endotracheal intubation was successful in 63.5% of the cases. I submit that that is a worse case probability, a worse case situation, because these subjects did not have tight policing of what they were doing.

In our own program, we approach a 90% to 95% success rate for our paramedics doing endotracheal intubation in the field. The training our people get is probably around 12 hours in that skill.

Conclusions

There is no question that endotracheal intubation is a superior airway control technique. I think also that the EGTA and EOA are certainly excellent devices. I do think that they represent a breakthrough. One must think about what one is doing, how one is doing it, what training feasibility is and the goals one is trying to attain.

Self-Evaluation Quiz

1. The components of airway control described in this paper are oxygenation, ventilation and aspiration protection.
   a) True
   b) False
2. Tracheal intubation generally provides a more ideal airway than the esophageal obturator airway.
   a) True
   b) False
3. Large numbers of rescue personnel can be trained in tracheal intubation.
   a) True
   b) False
4. Training large numbers of personnel in esophageal airway use is more feasible than training large numbers of personnel in tracheal intubation because:
   a) There are more esophageal airways than endotracheal tubes
   b) Less time is required to achieve an acceptable level of competence in tracheal intubation
   c) Less time is required to achieve an acceptable level of competence in esophageal airway use
   d) None of the above
5. The esophagogastric tube airway provides protection from aspiration of blood in patients with massive facial injury.
   a) True
   b) False

6. The esophagogastric tube airway provides protection from aspiration of gastric contents in patients with penetrating abdominal injuries.
   a) True
   b) False
7. The best way generally to improve oxygenation in patients in the field rescue situation is by using (an):
   a) Esophagogastric tube
   b) Mouth-to-mouth ventilation
   c) Endotracheal tube
   d) Increased inspired oxygen concentration
8. The esophagogastric tube airway is always totally free of complications.
   a) True
   b) False

Answers on page 289.

Medical Anti-Shock Trouser: A Pneumatic Device for the Treatment of Shock

Mary Beth Skelton, R.N.

Objectives

1. To describe the indications and contraindications for use of the MAST suit.
2. To describe the application of the MAST suit and the effects observed in the patient after application.
3. To describe the indications and procedure for removal of the MAST suit.

The Medical Anti-Shock Trousers (MAST) garment is being utilized both as a pre- and inhospital device for the treatment of shock. Elsewhere in this volume Dr. Benson addressed the priorities of initial assessment in trauma. He mentioned that a primary objective in airway maintenance is oxygenation. This is achieved by external and internal respiration. By providing a patent airway, adequate external respiration is usually provided. Oxygen is delivered to the alveoli where it crosses over the alveolar membrane and is picked up by the capillaries and circulated into the tissues.

Internal respiration refers to that part of the respiratory process by which we get the tissues oxygenated. In order to do this, according to the Fick principle, we must have adequate cardiac output and an adequate arterial-venous oxygen difference. If either one of these is insufficient as in various forms of shock, adequate tissue oxygenation will not be provided.

Mary Beth Skelton, R.N., Director of Paramedic Training, Department of Surgery, Tulane University School of Medicine, New Orleans, La.; Member, Board of Directors, American Trauma Society.

When presented with a patient who is in shock, there is a responsibility to try to correct that shock.

In the early part of this century Crile determined that the patient in shock should be assisted in getting adequate blood to the central circulation. This could be achieved if there was some type of device applied to the lower extremities and abdomen to push blood up into the central circulation. The application of a pneumatic device did not work at that time because he was applying his device to the chronically hypotensive rather than to the acutely hypotensive patient.

At the time of World War II, there was the problem of pilots fainting when they would go into deep spins or nose dives. The vessels in their lower extremities would vasodilate and pull the blood from the brain. They would faint and the aircraft would crash. Based on research done by Crile, the G-suit was developed. This provided pressure to the lower extremities and abdomen to push blood up into the central circulation to prevent fainting.

During the Vietnam War, there were many abdominal and lower extremity injuries from shrapnel and land mines. The G-suit was modified into what was called the Military Anti-Shock Trouser (MAST suit). This provided some form of stabilization for those experiencing abdominal and lower extremity injuries to get them to field hospitals with some form of blood pressure and to keep heart, brain and lung circulation at an adequate level during transport.

This device has now been adapted for use in an emergency situation to assist the shocky patient when blood or intravenous fluid is unavailable in adequate amounts to restore blood volume. It is now known as the Medical Anti-Shock Trouser (MAST suit).

The purpose of the MAST suit is to mobilize excess blood from the lower extremities and abdomen and return it up into the central triangle of circulation — heart, brain and lungs. Since this is a form of autotransfusion, the blood does not need to be typed or cross-matched. It has good oxygen-carrying capacity. The MAST suit also has the additional advantages, being a pneumatic device, of controlling hemorrhage from lacerations and also of stabilizing fractures of the pelvis and, to some extent, of the femur.

The indications for use of the MAST suit are as follows: (1) In patients with a systolic blood pressure below 100 mm Hg, when a shocklike state exists. A shocklike state may be assessed when there is tachycardia, poor brain perfusion, as evidenced by dizziness and decreased level of consciousness. (2) In patients who have bleeding wounds either of the lower extremities or of the abdomen. The bleeding can be tamponaded by inflation of the MAST suit. (3) In patients with pelvic fractures who are shocky from blood loss. Femur fractures can be immobilized partially with application of the MAST suit, but concurrent use of traction splint is recommended. (4) In patients with neurogenic shock. Treating neurogenic shock, especially in the pre-hospital phase without advanced life support capabilities, is difficult. The MAST suit will mobilize the blood pooled in the venous side of the circulatory system.

The only contraindication for use of the MAST suit is pulmonary edema.

The procedure for inflation of the MAST suit is as follows: (1) Check the blood pressure and obtain a baseline reading of the blood pressure. (2) Move the patient onto the pneumatic MAST suit either by sliding the MAST suit underneath the patient, protecting the spine, or log-rolling the patient onto the MAST suit. (3) Encase the lower extremities and the abdomen in the MAST suit and secure the Velcro straps. The way in which this particular device is designed, ease of application occurs if one applies the MAST suit to the patient's left leg first, the right leg second and the abdomen last. (4) Connect the foot pump and hoses to all of the appropriate compartments and proceed with inflation, pressing on the foot pump. Once inflation of the MAST suit begins, the blood pressure of the patient needs to be checked almost continuously. (5) When the patient's systolic blood pressure reaches approximately 100 to 110 mm Hg, stop inflation and close the stopcocks. Over-inflation is prevented by the pop-off valves and the slipping of the Velcro straps.

The internal pressure of the MAST suit will not exceed 104 mm Hg. If overinflation starts to occur, the pop-off valves activate and air is released to bring the internal pressure of the MAST suit back down to 104 mm Hg.

The patient's blood pressure needs to be monitored closely during application because in a healthy young person the pressure can frequently go up to 150 to 160 mm Hg systolic pressure. This may not be desired because of other injuries sustained, such as head trauma. An old contraindication for application of the MAST suit still found in the literature is an isolated head injury. If the patient is in shock and the only injury seen is a head injury, something else has to be occurring. He either has hidden bleeding in the thorax or abdomen due to ruptured viscus or may possibly be in neurogenic shock secondary to spinal cord trauma or massive intracranial pressure with herniation of the brain stem.

Research has been done indicating that use of the MAST suit to raise the systolic blood pressure to 100 to 110 mm Hg will not increase the intracranial pressure enough to further damage the brain. It will be enough, however, to provide perfusion to the kidneys, heart, brain and lungs, which is the objective in these patients.

The MAST suit should not be removed until proper fluid replacement is instituted and until surgical capabilities are available for that patient. If the MAST suit is removed prematurely, the fluid mobilized initially from the lower extremities and abdomen will return to those areas, sending the patient back into shock.

The procedure for deflation is as follows: (1) Check the patient's blood pressure. (2) Disconnect the tubes from the foot pump. (3) Open the stopcock of the abdominal compartment. (4) Recheck the blood pressure. (5) If there is a 5 mm Hg drop in the patient's blood pressure, stop deflation. (6) Increase IV fluid administration until the blood pressure recovers to the previous level. (7) Proceed with deflation. It may take 20 to 30 minutes to remove the MAST suit. If intra-abdominal hemorrhage is suspected, the MAST suit deflation should be accomplished in the operating room so that one has immediate surgical capabilities to handle the emergency.

What type of effects can be expected with application of the MAST? When the MAST suit is applied, perfusion is increased to the lungs. Alveolar wall ischemia is reduced. The capillary cell wall damage that is seen in shock is also reduced. When this occurs, the capillary permeability lessens. The baroreceptor response seen in shock is less, because the blood pressure is increased and the body does not have to compensate for the shocklike situation. Also, by providing an autotransfusion to the central circulation in the immediate, definitive treatment of the patient, less crystalloid and nonblood fluid has to be used in that initial resuscitation. Therefore, the total result is less effusion of fluid into the alveolar wall edema. One of the problems that we frequently see in a shock patient who has massive fluid resuscitation is adult respiratory distress syndrome (ARDS). We do not see a high incidence of this complication with the use of the MAST suit.

Following are some case histories demonstrating use of the MAST suit. In the first case, paramedics responded to a call that was diagnosed as a possible ectopic pregnancy. The woman was 27 years of age. When the paramedics arrived at the scene, her blood pressure was 0/0. They applied the MAST suit and her blood pressure immediately increased to 50/0. At this time, they started the IV fluids, which they were unable to do initially because of low blood pressure and peripheral vascular collapse. The MAST suit increased the perfusion to the upper extremities to such a degree that they were able to find the vein, get a large-bore needle inserted and an IV drip going. The woman received 2,000 ml of lactated Ringer's. On her admission to the emergency department her blood pressure was 100/60, at which time additional fluid resuscitation was begun. At the time the MAST suit was removed, she had a stable blood pressure of 120/70.

Hemoglobin was 8.2 and hematocrit was 26.8. She had lost a large amount of blood. She was taken to the operating room where a laparotomy was performed; 2,700 ml of blood was found in the abdominal cavity. She recovered with no complications and was dismissed from the hospital.

The second case history demonstrates that one can use the MAST suit for an injury above the level of the MAST suit. A 17-year-old man sustained a gunshot wound to the fourth intercostal space. When the paramedic unit arrived, his blood pressure was 70/0 and his condition was deteriorating rapidly. His blood pressure fell to 60/0. The MAST suit was applied, and his blood pressure increased to 90/0. In the emergency department chest tubes were inserted; 1,600 ml of blood was lost through the chest tubes. He was taken to the operating room. At that time, fluid resuscitation had been accomplished and, with the MAST suit still inflated, his blood pressure was found to be 170/70. The deflation process of the MAST suit was accomplished and he maintained a stable blood pressure of 120/80. His estimated blood loss was 4,500 ml of blood, which is just about an adult's total circulating volume.

There was a study done in the Kansas City area about two years ago in which 46 patients who had the MAST suit applied were evaluated. The initial blood pressure in 17 was below 50 mm Hg. In 17 patients, the initial pressure was between 50 and 80 mm Hg and in 12 patients the initial blood pressure was a little above 80 mm Hg. The MAST suit was applied to them all.

The initial pressure increase in 16 was 0 to 40, which means that they had an increase of 40 mm Hg over their initial pressure. Sixteen of these patients had a response of 40 to 80 mm Hg pressure, and six patients had a pressure response of greater than 80 mm Hg. Averaged out, there was an increase of 61 mm Hg in pressure immediately after application of the MAST suit. After arrival in the emergency department, the average pressure had risen to 75 mm Hg once fluid resuscitation was begun. After stabilization of the individual and removal of the MAST suit the average blood pressure was up 95 mm Hg.

What are some of the problems seen with the use of the MAST suit? There is some compromise in diaphragmatic excursion because of the abdominal contents pushing up against the diaphragm. A series done at the University of Kansas on arterial blood gases in patients with the MAST suit applied showed the oxygenation of the arterial blood was not adversely affected. The application of the MAST suit does compromise diaphragmatic excursion, but not to the extent that it prevents good oxygenation of the arterial blood.

The second problem is an increase in lactic acid production accompanied by an increase in the serum potassium. A research project was done on animals to study this. In the group of dogs in which the MAST suit pressure exceeded the dog's systolic pressure, increased lactic acid was produced which caused a lower blood pH. In the group of dogs in which the pressure of the MAST suit did not exceed the dog's systolic pressure, there was no evidence of acidosis.

Blood taken from both a peripheral and a femoral vein showed an increase in the serum potassium which was higher in those dogs in which the MAST suit pressure was higher than the dog's systolic pressure. Therefore, an increase in the production of anaerobic products, such as lactic acid, and potassium was seen when the MAST suit was applied to the dogs, especially when the pressure of the suit exceeded the systolic blood pressure. Consequently, it may result in a more profound systemic lacticacidosis and hyperkalemia, when the MAST suit is deflated. This may be treated by giving a bolus of sodium bicarbonate either immediately prior to or after the deflation of the MAST suit.

In conclusion, the use of the MAST suit is an innovative way to manage patients in shock both in the pre-hospital phase and in the emergency department until proper fluid replacement can be achieved. It is a means of stabilizing patients until the injuries producing the shock can be surgically managed.

Self-Evaluation Quiz

1. In which of the following situations is the use of the MAST suit indicated?
   a) Suspected intra-abdominal hemorrhage
   b) Open fracture of the femur with accompanied hemorrhage
   c) Severe shock from any cause
   d) Pulmonary edema
   e) a and c
   f) b and d
   g) a, b and c
   h) b, c and d
2. The MAST suit is applied in cases of hypovolemic shock because it:
   a) Decreases urinary output
   b) Increases diaphragm movement and aids breathing
   c) Provides an autotransfusion to the upper body
   d) Decreases the probability of acidosis in the lower extremities
3. When should the MAST suit be deflated?
   a) When the patient's vital signs are stable
   b) When hospital personnel need to take x-rays
   c) When fluid replacement can be performed for monitoring the patient's vital signs

d) When the patient must be examined by the triage nurse
e) a
f) b and d
g) a and c
h) c and d

4. At what point will the pop-off valves release excess pressure?
   a) 80 mm Hg
   b) 100 mm Hg
   c) 104 mm Hg
   d) 110 mm Hg
5. The MAST suit should be pumped up only until the systolic blood pressure of the patient reaches 100 to 110 mm Hg in head injured patients.
   a) True
   b) False
6. With the application of the MAST suit there is an increased incidence of the patient developing adult respiratory distress syndrome.
   a) True
   b) False
7. The MAST suit may be used to splint pelvic fractures complicated by shock.
   a) True
   b) False

Answers on page 289.

Family, Bystanders and Untrained Responders

Lawrence M. Hatfield, Jr., REMT

Objectives

1. To describe different ways the EMT can incorporate training of handling the trauma scene in their training programs.
2. To define different ways of handling the problems that the EMT can encounter in dealing with (a) bystanders, (b) first responders and (c) relatives.

Introduction

In the training programs for the emergency medical technician (EMT), both basic and advanced level, much improvement has been made and great strides have been taken in providing the proper training and skills necessary to allow pre-hospital personnel to provide the highest possible care for the victims of sudden onset illness or trauma. As training programs have continued to improve, so have the skill and the knowledge levels of our EMTs. However, there is one area which has been for the most part grossly neglected and, in the majority of cases unfortunately, has left EMTs improperly trained and ill-prepared to deal with the trauma situation — namely, the untrained responder or bystander, the first responders and the family or immediate relatives of the injured or ill patient.

To this end, much discussion and many new ideas have been forthcoming to more adequately prepare our EMTs for this problem. Some of these include case histories, group discussions

Lawrence M. Hatfield, Jr., REMT, Chairman, Society of EMT Instructor/Coordinators, NAEMT, Newton Highlands, Mass.

with family members of previously treated trauma or medically ill patients and, in some cases, role-playing, to more adequately prepare EMTs for their tasks. These new ideas, at the minimum, have greatly benefited the EMT, but in some cases have failed to go far enough or in sufficient depth to provide the EMT the knowledge he requires. Unfortunately, the old cliche "a little knowledge is a dangerous thing" more than aptly applies here, in that an EMT who has enough knowledge to handle a given situation in a given circumstance will be unable to cope with and respond appropriately and adequately to that unexpected situation which confronts him in a life-and-death crisis management situation.

Untrained Bystander

As alluded to earlier, we have three basic classes of individuals by whom we will be confronted at the scene of a sudden illness or trauma. The first is the untrained bystander or the individual who is at the scene, or arrives very shortly thereafter, of the sudden illness or injury who initiates what he feels to be appropriate and necessary care for the stricken individual. At times, these individuals are trained in first aid. However, in most cases, they have had no training but they feel the need to react or, in some cases, to overreact because of the situation and attempt to provide care for the patient. Upon arrival, the EMT will certainly have many problems, but he must be prepared to deal with this individual upon initial arrival.

To physically push him aside or order him out of the way does little to give this individual any feeling of self-satisfaction or esteem for attempting to care for the sick or injured person. Rather, the EMT should approach the individual, identify himself and then question the individual while assessing the patient. Many questions can be asked and much valuable information can be derived by speaking to the untrained bystander to ascertain whether the patient was breathing, has stopped breathing since he arrived, the amount and severity of bleeding which has occurred, how long since the onset of illness or injury, and what care if any this person has rendered to the patient.

This will often allow the EMT to better initiate his care and more adequately and properly treat the patient, because this is all *necessary information* which the hospital needs and which all well-trained EMTs will endeavor to obtain upon initiating treatment. Certainly, the adequacy of the information given can be determined by the qualified EMT as well by questioning the patient, if appropriate, and verifying again the information presented.

In crucial life-and-death situations, this untrained bystander often can be a great help to the EMT, the extra hands which we so frequently need for the holding of a flashlight, IV solutions, help in applying splinting materials or bandaging materials and, most importantly, in the case of the extremely anxious patient, that comforting glance and reassuring holding of the patient's hand.

First Responder

The second person the EMT may often encounter at the scene of a sudden illness or injury, and oftentimes the same as the bystander, is the first responder. For the purpose of this discussion we shall define the first responder as that individual who is dispatched to the scene and arrives prior to the ambulance and prior to the trained EMT. This individual can be the police officer, state highway patrolman, local fire fighter or a lesser trained and qualified individual, such as a person who has had American Red Cross first aid training only at the basic level or similar courses. Generally, we refer to the first responder as the individual who has a lesser degree of training than the EMT-A or the EMT-P.

Often, the first responder can be our greatest asset or our greatest liability at the scene, depending upon two factors: (1) the attitude of the first responder himself, whether he feels he has all the training necessary and whether he resents other individuals interfering when he has initiated patient care and (2) the attitude of the EMT and the way in which he approaches the first responder.

Approaching the first responder in a derogatory or demeaning manner certainly will create hostility to you and to EMTs in general. He may refuse to help you or even to give necessary and pertinent information.

The first responder's own attitude is generally one of the greatest concerns which we have at the scene. We all know and are aware that for years the American Red Cross first aid-trained ambulance attendant was all we had. Even ambulance attendants who had this level of training were often far and few between. As the state of the art grew and advanced, the EMT emerged upon the scene.

These veterans of the early ambulance services were frequently pushed aside, overlooked and were not given a chance to become a part of the new EMS system. Additionally, some of these individuals could neither grasp nor handle the EMT knowledge levels required and, therefore, were unable to obtain the coveted EMT patch. However, they generally had the sincerity and the desire to do what they could with the limited training they had. It is unfortunate that these individuals have been ignored or excluded from the EMS system by the young EMT who feels he knows it all. While their levels of training and knowledge may not be comparable to those of the EMT, most of these veterans have a streetwise knowledge that often surpasses the textbook knowledge of the EMT.

These veterans know how to deal with people as people whereas EMTs may often deal with a victim or a patient as an inanimate object, without feeling, without compassion, without understanding or emotion.

I have personally observed these veteran first responders at the scene who have been excellent in terms of dealing with the emotionally strained and disturbed patient. They exhibit a strong, secure, often strange sense of security to that individual or to the family. They have been handling ambulance calls for years. Many of them certainly know how to treat simple hemorrhage, manage airways, give cardiopulmonary resuscitation, help apply splints, load and transport patients.

It is truly detrimental to push aside this veteran first responder and not make adequate use of his skills. We often learn and benefit from these individuals. They are more than willing to help us, if we will only give them the chance.

The second part of this problem is that of the EMT and his attitude. As stated previously, the state of the art has changed. EMTs have become in many cases almost too well acclaimed and in some cases almost worshipped to the point that they feel that they are the only individuals who can treat a sick or injured patient. Unfortunately, I have seen EMTs who are not afraid to proclaim this attitude to the rest of the world.

This individual hurts not only the cause of EMS but all of us who are EMTs. He often provides inadequate and improper patient care because of his attitude. He will ridicule the old veteran first responder, the old first-aider and will not give him a chance to be a part of the system. They often fail to give due credit to these first responders, who may very well have kept a patient alive by giving artificial ventilation, closed chest heart massage, keeping the patient from exsanguinating by controlling hemorrhage or reducing the anxiety and the aggravation of injuries of the injured patient by their calm, reassuring look and the way in which they impart this to the patient or the victim at the scene.

It is most unfortunate when an EMT belittles this first responder and, in some cases, actually orders him away from the patient or shoves him aside when he arrives and announces to the world, perhaps by attitude only and not verbally, that the EMT is now on the scene and everything is going to be fine. It behooves every EMT, both new and experienced, to pay attention to the veteran first responder and learn from him. Their knowledge and capabilities in most cases are greatly needed by all of us and can make our jobs much easier, because they have mastered all the little tricks of the trade which new EMTs do not learn in the classroom, do not learn in the clinical setting, but acquire only after many ambulance calls and many hours of patient contact and patient care.

Relatives

The third individual the EMT will deal with is the immediate relative or immediate family member of the patient. If not properly handled, this person can be your greatest problem, much more of a problem than the patient for whom you are caring. The family member will see his loved one lying there in the street, sick or appearing to be very badly injured, and he is not interested at that point in the gravity of the situation but, rather, in transporting the patient to a hospital for definitive care.

We have made significant strides in public education of what the EMT is and the pre-hospital emergency room on wheels concept, but we still have a long way to go. Family members are often the first to forget this when it involves a loved one. The

EMT should react even more professionally, deal with the situation more than appropriately and make every effort to project himself as the professional he truly is.

How do we deal with the emotionally uncontrollable, highly anxious relative? There is no easy answer. The best way is with a reassuring look, the commanding voice which says to the patient and family member that you know what you are doing and are in control of the situation. Despite the butterflies in the stomach, the nausea, the awfulness of seeing somebody die, this image must prevail and emanate from the EMT, because if you cannot control yourself at the scene, you cannot control the family member and you cannot care for your patient. By exhibiting a strong sense of command and an air of competency, and by having the situation in hand, you will immediately convey this to the family member, who will probably respond appropriately by becoming more controllable, at least to the point where you can talk to and reassure him. This is not to say that it will work every time. Many times it will not. On occasion, it will be necessary for you to become very commanding. By that I do not mean dictating or domineering, but you must be in command, in control. If you cannot deal with the family, you cannot deal with your patient.

We talked earlier about first responders. They are often the most qualified at the scene to deal with the family member, the emotionally upset, the highly nervous, distraught, disturbed, anxious patient. If you have a first responder at the scene, ask him to deal with the family member. Do not ignore or push aside relatives. The family member must be cared for, just as the patient must be cared for. If the first responder is having trouble with the family member, go to them when appropriate and lend your reassurance to put the situation in control and then return to your patient.

What happens if you do not have a first responder and the relative is yelling or crying and pulling at you? In some cases relatives will even try to take patient care equipment from the patient. Again, you must be firm but fair with this individual and put him to work. Do not let him idly watch while you are caring for the patient. If you can, have him get with the family on the other side and talk to the patient as well as the family member. Have him hold his loved one's hand. Have him help you. Give him something to hold; I do not care if it is a bottle of lactated Ringer's. It keeps him occupied. Communicate and talk, tell him what you are going to do, if you are going to splint the leg or if you are going to put on a cervical collar, and why you are doing it. For example, do not tell him a leg is broken, but rather you think the leg may be broken and you want to protect it so the injury does not worsen. Do it in a way that will instill confidence.

Sometimes available to help you at the scene of an accident is a member of the clergy — a priest, rabbi, minister or other member of the church. They often will come forward to you, identify themselves readily and ask if they can be of any assistance. They are not offering assistance in providing patient care. Rather, they want to help with the emotional problem of the patient or the anxiety of the family member. Use this asset if it is available to you. As veteran first responders, they often have the training and ability to deal with accident victims or family members far and above that which EMTs have received. Use them in your pre-hospital care setting as appropriate.

One of the greatest problems with which EMTs and people in EMS have to deal is what to do with the family member when it is time to transport the patient to the hospital. Where do you put him — in the front seat or in the back of the ambulance? Do you ask him to go to the hospital in his own vehicle or ask the police officer to bring him to the hospital? There is no rule. This is a judgment situation and it must be dealt with on each case's merits. In the absence of regulations or policies which prohibit family members from the ambulance, do whatever is appropriate at the time. If the trauma victim is a 3-year-old child, do not try to put the child in the back of the ambulance without the mother of the child. You will have more of a problem. Get the mother under contol and put her in the back of the ambulance with the child because the child wants it that way. The child will not respond to you without her mother with her.

Use your judgment. If the child is very seriously ill or hurt, if the child is close to death, you had better deal with the parent in an appropriate way. Put the parent with a police officer or another crew member and get them away from your ambulance.

Personally, I do not like to have anybody in the back of my ambulance unless I am dealing with a small child, because if the patient suffers sudden death, then you have two people to cope with. In the back of the ambulance, you do not have time to deal with two people. You only have time to deal with one person — the patient.

However, be sure that you have the family member under control if you put him in the ambulance, and this applies to the front as well as the back, because if the family member is in the front seat, all he will hear is the siren wailing, he will visualize the ambulance, see what is going on in the back, look through the window, if he possibly can. If he hears the radio communications or that things in the back are going badly, he is going to react.

Conclusion

The manner in which the EMT handles the untrained bystander, first responder and family member has a very significant and profound impact upon the patient care given at the scene. As professional EMTs, we are expected to be held accountable for the care which we give to the victim. We talked earlier of ways to achieve this during training. I wish to emphasize this area, as with other areas of EMT training, must be continually upgraded and grown or expanded upon. No EMT I have ever observed or taught or worked with at either level has ever demonstrated that after six hours in a classroom he has learned how to cope with an emotionally disturbed patient or an emotionally disturbed family member. As with all aspects of EMS, the laboratory sessions and, in this particular instance, I am talking about role-playing, bringing in family members from previous calls, bringing in the victim himself, if you establish a rapport with them — this is the only way in which you will learn to handle these situations. It must not stop there. You must not quit upon graduation and the wearing of the EMT patch or pin. You cannot be expected and you must never feel that you know it all, in any aspect of EMS, particularly this area which we have overlooked in our training programs until recently. The EMT who subscribes to this philosophy clearly cheats himself and, unfortunately and most dramatically, the patient in the field. To that end he is detrimental to our cause as EMTs.

Self-Evaluation Quiz

1. In acquiring all necessary knowledge about dealing with the relatives of injured or sick patients the EMT needs to remember:
   a) Only that which he learned during his formal training
   b) To learn from each case because each is different and will add to his knowledge
   c) To establish his own set of rules for handling all cases and never deviate
   d) To forget all knowledge since there will always be someone else present to deal with the problem
2. One of the best ways to handle relatives at the scene of a medical emergency is to:
   a) Give them something to do to help you because this keeps them occupied and easier to handle
   b) Have a police officer remove them from the scene as quickly as possible
   c) It doesn't really matter what you do with relatives because they will always be uncontrollable
3. The EMT, upon arriving at the scene at which a bystander is with the patient, should:
   a) Immediately order him away from the patient
   b) Ask and obtain all pertinent and necessary information about the patient and what if anything this person has done for him
   c) Advise the bystander that he is covered by the Good Samaritan law
   d) Advise the bystander that he should never interfere again because he can be held accountable for injury to the patient
4. First responders may be one of the greatest assets an EMT can have, but the EMT must remember that some first responders may:
   a) Be uncooperative because they are jealous and untrusting of the EMT
   b) Be helpful in treating the patient but only to the level of their training and knowledge

c) Not want to give up the care of the patient to the EMT
d) All of the above

5. The single biggest *immediate* asset the EMT has at the scene of an emergency is the:
   a) Physician on the radio
   b) Patient
   c) Willing bystander
   d) Ability to recognize those life-threatening emergencies and treat them accordingly
6. The one factor which has often been said to distinguish first responders from the EMT is:
   a) EMTs will often deal with patients as inanimate objects while the first responder deals with the patient as a person respecting his feelings and emotions
   b) EMTs will deal with the patient regarding his feelings and emotions while the first responders deal with the patients as inanimate objects
   c) EMTs and first responders both deal with patients as individuals
   d) There is no difference between the way in which both groups deal with patients
7. The EMT must always remember that the most important thing to the family member at the scene of the emergency is:
   a) Transportation to the hospital for definitive care
   b) Care to be given at the scene
   c) The knowledge of the EMT
   d) How long the family member will be in the hospital

Answers on page 289.

Hazardous Substances

David Whisenhunt

Objectives

1. To discuss methods of identifying hazardous materials in transit.
2. To identify agencies which can provide assistance and information during emergencies.

In the case of emergency medical technicians responding to an accident involving hazardous substances, if there are fire protection and law enforcement personnel already at the scene they will take whatever precautions necessary to evacuate people, cordon off the area and keep spectators away. They will probably have most of the problems solved before you get there. However, if you are first at the scene, what do you do? You are not going to have much time. Unfortunately, we do not have an ironclad answer to this problem.

There are three means of identifying shipments of hazardous materials: (1) placards, (2) shipping papers and (3) labels and marking on the containers. These are the three methods that EMTs, fire protection personnel, law enforcement officials and the public have of identifying hazardous materials.

Placards are diamond-shaped signs appearing on tractor trailers, railroad cars and cargo tanks. These identify the class of hazardous material and tell you what the hazard is — for example, explosives. If there is a diamond-shaped placard on a vehicle that says explosives, it is more than likely going to be dynamite or some other explosive compound comparable to dynamite.

Vehicles now have shipping papers with the driver in the driver's compartment. They should either be in the driver's suit

---

David Whisenhunt, Lieutenant, Georgia State Patrol, Department of Public Safety, Atlanta, Ga.

or around the door, but they are required to be within his reach. The containers themselves should also be marked and labeled.

In the case of explosives and a fire, the recommendation is to evacuate the area. If you were responding to a similar incident and were the first on the scene, what should you do if there are injuries? It is going to be your decision.

If the fire can be contained, and if it is not in the area of the cargo, you probably have a little time. If the fire has already reached the cargo when you arrive at the scene, you are operating on borrowed time.

However, if the fire and law enforcement officials are already there, they should take the proper precautions. They will assist you in your attempts to treat the injured. But, if you are the first one at the scene, you are going to have a problem. Some people say that due to the fire and smoke, they could not see the placard. So you never know what you are going to have in any particular situation until you arrive at the scene.

In addition to explosives, there are many other classes of hazardous materials with which you should be familiar, for example, poisons.

Let me give you details of an accident involving poisons. A truck contained 20 cylinders of methyl bromide. Methyl bromide is an insecticide, a poison and, in this case, it was a gas. These 20 cylinders contained 2,000 lb of methyl bromide, 98% and 2% chloral pitrin. Chloral pitrin is a poisonous irritant which was put in with the methyl bromide to provide an odor so that escaping gas could be detected more readily. So we had a poisonous gas. The truck collided with a car containing eight occupants. Cylinders went through the forward compartment of the trailer. Some cylinders ruptured, and they blended their gases and escaped into the atmosphere. Four of the occupants of the car left the scene under their own power. The driver of the truck left the scene. In the immediate area around the truck cab and the vehicle there was some debris. These containers were scattered about and gas was escaping. Four occupants of the vehicle never left the scene. One bystander removed a young lady across the road, but, unfortunately, the area to which the bystander removed the victim was still in the vicinity of the escaping gas. When a state trooper arrived on the scene, the driver told him that he had poison gas in his cargo. The trooper saw the gas venting from the cylinders and called the fire department. This was just prior to meeting the driver of the truck and the trooper thought it was smoke. So the fire department responded. The driver could not provide the trooper with information other than that he was transporting gas. He did not know the characteristics of the gas or what precautions to take. He had a chemical company identifying card in the cab of the truck, but he did not even give him that information.

As a result of this accident, four of the passengers of the vehicle died from poisoning. The state trooper and some spectators were exposed to it and treated. Altogether, there were four fatalities and approximately 40 injuries — 40 people treated for gas inhalation! This is just an example of what can happen. The vehicle was placarded, but it would not make any difference to me if I was to encounter what they call poison A or poison B. A poison is a poison! If you are responding to an accident similar to this one, you need to know what you are dealing with and what precautions you should take, how to protect yourself and others at the scene.

There are many other classes of hazardous materials, such as oxidizers. Oxidizers decompose very rapidly to yield oxygen. In combination with other chemicals, they can be explosive.

There are also radioactive materials, classes 1, 2 and 3. If I were to feel comfortable at all with hazardous materials, I think I would feel most comfortable handling radioactive materials because regulations pertaining to the packaging, marking and transportation of radioactive materials are probably the strictest of all hazardous materials being transported today. I do not think they have had one fatality from exposure due to the transportation of radioactive materials.

There are some agencies that can assist you when you are responding to an accident involving hazardous materials. They will provide the expertise that you need to handle the situation. Some of you are probably already aware of these agencies and the kinds of services they provide. But we cannot all be experts in the field of transportation of hazardous materials. The most important thing to know is how to identify them and who can assist you.

The Chemical Transportation Emergency Center (CTEC), a chemical manufacturers association, provides 24-hour service.

They have a toll-free telephone number (800/424-9300). If you call them from the scene of an accident, they will want to know certain information:

1. Name of the caller and your call-back number. They do not want you to call, then hang up and leave the phone because they are going to call you back in a very short time.
2. Location of the problem.
3. Name of the shipper or manufacturer of the product being transported. You will need to obtain this information from the shipping papers unless you can talk to the driver.
4. Type of container if the product is in containers.
5. Name of the carrier who is performing the transportation.
6. Consignee's name, where it is going.
7. Local conditions at the scene of the accident.

When you provide this information, they will tell you what precautions to take at the scene. This is only for emergency conditions. They will not tell you about physical and chemical properties of the product and its effects. They will only tell you what emergency measures to take. Hopefully, someone will already be there to handle this. But if you are the first person on the scene, it is your responsibility to take these precautions.

They will also provide you with information pertaining to materials other than chemicals. They have telephone contacts all over the United States. They have communications with other chemists. They will be able to provide you with information on who can assist you locally through their telephone contacts. This is the agency to contact when you are confronted with any chemical emergency.

The National Agricultural Chemical Association can provide you with personnel, equipment and expertise to clean up and decontaminate an accident scene. Their telephone number is (513)961-4300. They will provide you with information on any Class B poisons. There are over 2,000 poisons in Class B, mostly insecticides and herbicides. This agency will provide you with a service similar to CTEC.

For dealing with radioactive materials, there is a Department of Radioactivity in the Health Department in Georgia that has a goal team ready to assist you.

Although many of the dangers of transporting hazardous materials cannot be eliminated, they can be minimized through planning.

Self-Evaluation Quiz

1. Three methods of identifying hazardous materials are (a) placards, (b) shipping papers and (c) labels and marking.
   a) True
   b) False
2. In the case of explosives and fire, it is not necessary to evacuate the area.
   a) True
   b) False
3. Regulations pertaining to packaging, marking and transporting radioactive materials are the strictest of all hazardous materials.
   a) True
   b) False

Answers on page 289.

The Emergency Medical Services Communications System

Carl C. Van Cott

Objectives

At the end of this paper the reader should have a new perspective of EMS communications systems and be able to consider them in a broader context of a system of exchanges of information rather than in a strict radio or electronic context. The reader will recognize five common outline points as applied to EMS communications and be able to use these five points as an evaluation aid in assessing his own EMS communications system.

Introduction

Emergency medical service communications systems have evolved over a period of decades with a minimum of guidance or direction. Communications systems were fabricated to meet localized needs with a minimum of forethought applied to the overall total system requirement. EMS communications have been historically regarded as radio communications linkages between ambulance and hospital units. This paper attempts to consider more than just the ambulance treatment team to physician or hospital communication and strives to consider those functional communications linkages and exchanges required to interconnect the resources, manpower, vehicles and equipment required to address effectively the emergency medical response.

Carl C. Van Cott, Assistant Chief, North Carolina State Office of Emergency Medical Services, Communications and Engineering Branch, North Carolina Department of Human Resources, Division of Facility Services, Raleigh.

Emergency medical communication is a new and expanding discipline and, for the most part, is still little understood. Even an experienced communications engineer working in this field sometimes encounters difficulty with the medical terminology or expressions, federal funding agency requirements or new communications devices or communications needs. This is understandable because for the last several decades, EMS communications consisted primarily of installing radio transmitters in ambulances to allow the ambulance attendant to communicate to a hospital, or a radio in a rescue vehicle to allow the rescue squad to talk to their dispatcher. Radios for these systems were obtained and installed by various motivated groups or individuals from any number of sources, companies or other emergency service agencies, sometimes on a hand-me-down basis. Wide area compatibilities and functional usage of the resources seldom exist in these systems.

The relatively recent recognition of emergency medical services as a neglected area of health care and public service has generated a considerable amount of effort to strive and improve the communications mechanisms for the health care unit. For all of this interest and activity to be applied in an effective and productive manner, however, some plan or central guidance must be evident to allow the various evolving systems within an area to strive toward a common goal. It must be recognized that the communications service required by an ambulance, hospital or a medical community is interactive with the communications systems and community services around it. For purposes of this discussion, EMS communications will be considered to be those exchanges of information or ideas between the various individuals or response units necessary to coordinate or deliver emergency medical services to the public. This communications unit in turn becomes an integral part of a larger and more complicated communications function. Note that in this context, communication is not considered to be only radio or electronic communication, but considers all exchanges, both formal and informal, between the various provider service groups and the public.

Discussion

Let us first take inventory of the EMS resources within our system. In this discussion, we will consider the medical services within a geographical area such as a large city or county. These resources will vary according to locality and individual local requirements, but generally will consist of rescue squads (both volunteer and paid professional such as fire department units), ambulance services (municipality and privately operated) and other medical response units. This latter category can include public safety officers or "first response" units such as sometimes are operated by fire departments or law enforcement agencies. Additionally, our medical system includes the hospital community. This includes the fixed facilities, nurses, physicians and emergency department staff required for the effective delivery of medical service. These resources, then, constitute the majority of the required equipment, personnel and vehicles necessary to form the medical response unit. Let us now consider how these resources can be integrated with the other public services necessary for the functioning whole of public service.

During the delivery of emergency medical services, communications are often necessary between several diverse groups of people located at different places. For example, when an emergency incident occurs and is detected, someone must assess the situation and, upon determining the need for medical assistance, must report it to the medical resource delivery mechanism. After the emergency incident is reported, the EMS system must be able to dispatch and coordinate the manpower, vehicles and equipment required to totally respond to the situation. There must be trained individuals taking the calls for public assistance. These individuals must be capable of rapidly determining the type of emergency and the type of equipment or resources necessary to totally respond to that emergency. They must know the status and whereabouts of their resources at any given time in order to direct effectively the resource to the emergency, and they must be given communications linkages and ties with other public safety agencies, such as law enforcement and fire services, so these may be utilized effectively in the delivery of the service to the public.

After the medical treatment team has been dispatched and has arrived at the location of the emergency, the team must be able to communicate both with the coordinating body (the dispatcher) and the medical treatment facility (the hospital).

They must be able to assess the situation and, if necessary, call for additional resources or turn back superfluous resources that may already be enroute to the scene. Upon completing the at-scene treatment in preparation of transporting their patient, the ambulance team must be able to communicate with the hospital emergency department to alert or notify the hospital that they will be bringing a patient to the hospital location. This allows the hospital to prepare for reception of the patient and leads to better patient care and delivery of a more coordinated service. In advanced life support (ALS) or paramedic systems, there must be communications linkages established to allow the ambulance treatment team and the physician at a remote location to easily and rapidly exchange information to enable the delivery of advanced life support skills at the patient's location. These advanced life communications may require the application of radio EKG telemetry to allow the field paramedic team to transmit electrocardiograph information to the hospital. Telemetry transmission, however, is generally considered to be optional within the advanced life system, and determination for its inclusion in a system must be made on a local level in discussion with the directing physicians. It should be emphasized that the inclusion of sophisticated electronic mechanisms is not a substitute for the requisite training that must be given the paramedic. The radio telemetry is no more than a tool and, as such, must be used by a skilled artisan to be of any value.

Upon delivery of the patient to the medical facility, the ambulance crew must be able to report to the dispatcher that they are again available for service, thus completing the EMS resource delivery cycle.

By analyzing the above information transfers, it will be recognized that EMS communication may be broken into four general categories or aspects as follows:

1. Public access to the EMS resource delivery system.
2. Dispatch and coordination of the EMS resource.
3. Medical communication consisting of two levels of information exchange:
    a. Notification of hospital of the impending arrival of a patient, and

b. Advanced life support communications including the application of EKG telemetry where required.

4. Interagency communication.

Interagency communications are those exchanges necessary to coordinate with other public safety agencies within the geographic area of the system. These agencies include law enforcement, fire departments and the public utilities. EMS communications can be broken into one of the four above-listed categories. There is, however, a fifth category of EMS information exchange — communications education — which deals with the information exchanges necessary to impart the knowledge required to make the other parts of the system function: for example, the education of the public at large to use the established public access mechanism. Additionally, the education of the dispatchers or telecommunicators who receive the requests for emergency assistance is included in the fifth category as well as the aspects required to educate all members of the EMS team on the usage of their equipment and their role in the system. These, too, are EMS communications. The question, then, becomes one of how do all of the diverse resources become educated and coordinated into a functional unit?

One method that has been used for consolidating the EMS communications requirement is the establishment of the Central Medical Emergency Dispatch center, referred to as a CMED. The CMED serves as the receiving center for all medical emergency calls for the service area. A single telephone number is established and assigned to the CMED, thus consolidating the diversity of numbers required by the public to access the emergency medical services system. In most areas each individual rescue squad, ambulance service, fire department or other medical resource delivery mechanism, including the hospital, has its own telephone number listed in the telephone book. The public, when faced with a medical crisis or emergency, is confused as to which agency to call for assistance. By establishing only one well-publicized number, the time required for the access and response can be greatly reduced. The answering point or CMED will have communications linkages established to the other resources within the geographic area. These include telephone lines or radio transmission capabilities to each of the rescue squads and ambulance service providers, as well as mechanisms for radio alerting the volunteer members of these services. The CMED additionally has communications linkages to other public safety services, including law enforcement agencies and fire departments. This allows a coordinated response to be made by any of the emergency services. If an ambulance team needs fire department assistance, they may readily obtain this by communicating to the CMED and, in turn, relaying the information to the fire department. Should law enforcement for some reason be required, it may be obtained by contacting the CMED. Through the CMED the request is coordinated with the other responding agency.

For this coordinated effort response mechanism to be truly effective, it is necessary that a center be established for law enforcement and an additional center for fire protection communication. These three centers — the CMED, the central law enforcement dispatch center and the central fire emergency dispatch center — form the basis of what has been referred to as the triad of public safety. Each center is responsible for consolidating and coordinating their own respective resources within the geographic area. Conceivably, there will be three centers established: the CMED for medical, the CFED for fire and the CLED for law enforcement. These centers may be coincidental and located within the same physical plant or may be geographically dispersed throughout the service area if the necessary interconnecting communications are established. When taken to this level, it may be seen that there could easily be three telephone numbers for public access to the triad of public safety: one for fire, one for law enforcement and one for medical assistance. If this mechanism were in place, it would be a logical and recommended step to establish an emergency resource coordination center or public safety answering point (PSAP). This central answering point would publish one telephone number for access to all public safety agencies. Ultimately, the publicized telephone number would be 911, the three-digit national emergency telephone number.

Conclusions

From the above discussion, it may be seen that if all localities would structure their EMS communications around a standard model, a natural system compatibility would be developed that leads eventually to the availability of the nationally recognized emergency telephone number 911. It will additionally be recognized that by using a simple five-point outline consisting of (1) access, (2) dispatch and control, (3) medical communication, (4) interagency communication and (5) communication education and applying this outline on a local basis, the EMS communications system for an area may be assessed with the strong and weak points of the system becoming readily evident. These weak points may then be singled out for a concentrated effort for improvement, insuring the development of a well-rounded system design in which all five outlined points are eventually addressed.

Self-Evaluation Quiz

1. The elements of the triad of public safety are considered to be EMS, police and fire.
   a) True
   b) False
2. The Central Medical Emergency Dispatch center links the diverse resources required to respond to medical emergencies in a coordinated fashion.
   a) True
   b) False
3. EMS communications should be considered as those exchanges of information or ideas required to totally respond and coordinate the EMS resource delivery mechanism.
   a) True
   b) False
4. Five elements or aspects of EMS communications are public access, dispatch and coordination, medical communication, interagency communication and communications education.
   a) True
   b) False
5. EKG radio telemetry is considered as a necessity in all advanced life support (paramedic) systems.
   a) True
   b) False
6. When evaluating an EMS communications system using the five-point outline, if a weak point in the system is noted, it

should be corrected and improved without consideration being given to any of the other points.

a) True

b) False

Answers on page 289.

Medical Control: The Rural Experience

Ken Kimball, M.D.

Objectives

1. To recognize the importance of definitive state legislation that defines clearly the responsibilities, areas of authority and limitations of all involved in EMS.
2. To discuss ambulance right of way as opposed to traffic control by police.
3. To define and describe various aspects of medical control.

Regardless of the application of medical direction, we should think in terms of legal liability and legal permission. When there is going to be physician direction, it is imperative a good state law exists which defines what one may and may not do in order to avoid future difficulties. I shall not pursue that any further; however, I would caution you to be certain that you have a well-defined set of criteria under which to operate.

Some of our states already have laws governing paramedics, but many do not. This is an opportune time for us to work with our state legislators to see that there is a good law enacted. For example, in Nebraska it is a felony for anyone to claim he is a paramedic if he is not. A physician in a remote area should have a reasonable assurance that if someone says he is a paramedic that he is really dealing with someone who is trained. You should know the people with whom you are working and I think by and large we do. But if that circumstance were to arise, I think it is important that this be defined. We have to define what they may do simply on the basis that most of the states

---

Ken Kimball, M.D., Vice-Chairman, Committee on Trauma, American College of Surgeons, Kearney, Neb.; Founding Member, American Trauma Society.

wrote their medical practice acts back in the days when they said a physician may do so forth and so on and, therefore, by implication, no one else may do that unless there is a law that you may do it or you can do what you have been trained to do, as long as you are certified by the state and as long as it is done under the direction of a physician.

My point is: be sure of what you have. Many of us have had services operating illegally where the physician has accepted the responsibility, but I think there is no question that if there is not a state law allowing it, you are at risk and somebody is going to be caught. We should try to obtain good state legislation.

When we wrote our state law, it specifically stipulated that the paramedic may not be found guilty unless there is willful neglect. They have to not only prove that he did something wrong, but they also have to prove that he intended to do it. Likewise, the physician is held blameless as long as he makes reasonable medical judgments on the information that is provided to him. Again, documentation becomes important, but having a good state law is also important.

In an emergency people are going to do whatever they can, but the only thing we can really talk about is what may they legally do. I do not know of a single state in the United States that will legally allow an 81-hour EMT-A to do anything that is invasive, such as start IVs, do endotracheal intubation, insert chest tubes or defibrillate. I would hope they would do it to me if I were there under those circumstances, but it probably would not be legal. Some court would have to decide whether the law was set aside because it was an emergency situation.

Remember, the red light and siren do not give you the right of way; they let that vehicle request it. Be certain that your ambulance people understand that. We just had one ambulance destroyed recently because the driver thought he had the right of way. In modern vehicles, with the windows rolled up, the tape deck playing and the air conditioning on, it is difficult for people to see the red light or hear the siren. Many communities are no longer providing escorts to ambulances. Instead, when the ambulance calls in, if it goes through a center, they coordinate this with the police who stop traffic at major intersections. The problem with escort is that the police vehicle is ahead of you; he goes tearing down the street, motorists stop and let him go by and then they pull right out in front of the ambulance. So we are finding that it is a better approach in many communities to consider coordinating with the police, allow them to control traffic but not to actually escort the ambulance.

Remember that there are relatively few physicians in any one given area who have an interest in trauma, just as there are relatively few who have an interest in cardiology or in cancer or any other specialty. Sometimes, we become discouraged because we can find only three physicians out of 50 who really are interested in working to establish a system. I simply remind you that that is probably a lucky number if you can find three out of 50. Do not be discouraged, but try to identify the few who have a particular interest.

Historically, when we talk about physician control, most of us think in terms of the physician supervising the paramedic. If I may, I am going beyond that, and I shall suggest that medical control has to start with the development of the EMS council. The EMS council, which is going to really be the legal entity that controls the development of EMS in your local area, must have physician involvement. It should not be dominated by physicians, but there must be physician input.

The physician must be involved in the training of the ambulance attendant. That does not mean he has to teach all the classes, but he must know what is being done for several reasons: (1) he is going to want to have input as to what the particular procedure that is being taught to the EMT is going to be and (2) it is important that he know what these people have been trained to do, so that he can make maximum utilization of their capabilities. Most important, he is going to develop a rapport with these people with whom he will be talking periodically if he has an adequate communications system.

Physician control must involve the physician in a regular and a scheduled type of continuing education. The physician, the nurse, the ambulance attendant should all have regular meetings to critique the care that is being provided in that area. This is particularly true in a rural setting. One needs to talk about what was done well, what was done poorly and how one can do a better job of providing care for the patient.

Physician control has to involve consultation directly on a real-time basis with the ambulance attendant, whether the attendant is an EMT-A or an EMT-P. Obviously, if there is going to be paramedic operations, there must be a direct control of the operation of that individual by a physician at some point.

Rural groups have particular problems that relate to paramedic operation: (1) they do not have a big central hospital; (2) they often do not have full-time people in the hospital; and (3) they frequently have great distances involved. We have four counties in Nebraska that do not have even an ambulance service let alone a hospital or a physician or a paramedic operation. It may be 60, 80 or even 100 miles from some of the wilderness areas to a hospital that can provide care.

The converse is that there is probably no place in the world that needs a paramedic operation greater than do some of the rural areas. But then the problem is: How do you deal with this? How do you maintain these people as being competent? How do you insure direct interrelationship between the physician and the paramedic? We think this should be done by rotating the paramedics through a central hospital that is the control hospital where they work with the physicians who are going to be involved, talking to them on the two-way radio.

We think that physician control has to include refresher training courses. I am a great believer in the fact that refresher training is not the end of all ends. I often think of Dr. Farrington, who used to say that one should not let somebody make a mistake every day for two years and think of that as good experience. When we have a problem, we should identify it immediately or during the first week or month and should resolve it. Therefore, I am not strongly in favor of a refresher course every two years; I much more prefer physician input on a continuing education basis.

The backbone of this whole system is communications. The only point I would make at this time is that you should have communication centers that tie all of your emergency communication together. If you have that, then everybody can have his own radio frequency. There is no need for the physician to have a police radio or a national guard radio and a highway patrol radio. All he needs is his medical radio because if he can get into the center, they can interface him to any other frequency. They can cross-patch him to a telephone, they can put him into a conference group or whatever.

In a rural area of Nebraska, we put these units on the physician. They have touch-tone. The physician can access telephone line directly or he can go directly to the center. He can go to any hospital, talk to any ambulance, to the fire department, to the police department or to the national guard. Once he gets to the center, they simply cross-patch him.

On our EMS system we have selective paging, so that if I have my radio on, I can be called when I am in or out of town.

One thing that we have done that is rather unique, and I shall mention it only briefly. We have tied again all of our six centers together by dedicated lines. This is expensive. We have arranged to get the state to contract with the telephone company at government rates; they agree to provide the tie lines under a state contract. Therefore, we pay 70 cents a mile for our dedicated tie lines instead of $4 to $6 per mile. That is a substantial saving.

Second, by putting these units on the physician and by tying every hospital into the center, day to day, people use the system, and we charge the physician $25 to $50 per month for his service to use this. We charge the hospital approximately 50 cents per long distance call, and they can call anywhere in the United States on the system. That means that (1) the physician uses this daily and (2) the hospital uses the communications system that ties everything together daily.

We have three codes (1) code green, which means no priority; (2) code orange, which is something that is urgent but not emergency; and (3) code blue, which is emergency and takes everything else off the system.

Day to day the hospital is now using this for all of their communications. The average cost of a long distance call has decreased from $1.25 to 50 cents for the hospital. They are accustomed to using the system; yet, in times of emergency, we can wipe out the routine use and we have a dedicated established system that allows us to go across the state.

One must have a communications system as well as the dedicated physician who is tied to that system who will be available at a time of emergency.

Telemetry is important! Being from a rural area, I always become a little concerned, and I am going to talk the other way right now. I do not think there is any question that we should strive in our systems to have telemetry. You do not have to die just because you do not have telemetry. But do not let anyone get the idea that it is not helpful and that you really do not need to think about it. You should try to evolve a plan of telemetry in your system.

The same is true on passing local hospitals. We hear so frequently from the metropolitan area that all one needs to do is to rush patients into the big downtown center. I am really concerned that people think that they do not have to provide any care to the patient — all they need do is rush him to the big downtown hospital, as was done 20 years ago. If you are in a metropolitan area, if you have a preplanned program and you have identified hospitals that are trauma centers, coronary centers, and so forth, that is wonderful. Follow your protocol and take the victims where they are supposed to go. But if you are living in a rural area, you must go to the closest hospital and physician, stabilize the patient and then consider the transfer of that patient to another institution.

Good patient records are imperative.

I think there is a natural apprehension on the part of physicians and hospital administrators whenever anyone is going to do anything that can be documented. However, when they see the system function, they will appreciate that it is good protection. I think after it exists for a time, it is not any problem.

Self-Evaluation Quiz

1. In regard to ambulances, it is preferable to coordinate with the police, allowing them to control traffic rather than to escort.
   a) True
   b) False
2. The author favors physician input on a continuing basis rather than a refresher course every two years.
   a) True
   b) False
3. According to the author, telemetry is important and should be part of the EMS system.
   a) True
   b) False

Answers on page 289.

Observations on the Rural Aspects of an EMS System

Charles Aprahamian, M.D.

Objectives

1. To define and discuss urban-rural relationships as they relate to emergency medical care.
2. To discuss the development of the need for and the implications of urban-rural relationships.
3. To inform the reader of the direct effects and sequelae of indirect effects in terms of physician practice.

There is a familiar town-gown relationship which we all know about which makes reference to the integration of university medical philosophy and the daily practice of medicine. With the advent of EMS, there has been witnessed the development of an urban-rural relationship or what could be called the "rural connection." The purpose of this paper is to explore this connection and to give an example of how it may work.

"Rural" may be defined as referring to country people or life. It represents a community of less than 5,000 and is often characterized by a lack of a medical contingency. If a hospital is present, it will undoubtedly have community or basic hospital capabilities. "Urban" refers to, or is characteristic of, a city and has all the conveniences and nuisances associated with it. In this context, it represents a community with general or area hospital capability with or without a medical school affiliation. "Relationship" is defined as the state of being mutually or reciprocally interested, as in social, commercial or, for the purpose of this paper, patient care matters.

Charles Aprahamian, M.D., Assistant Professor of Surgery, Medical College of Wisconsin, Milwaukee.

In 1973 and again in 1976, a survey of hospital capabilities was carried out in Wisconsin. In the initial survey, teams of physicians, nurses, ambulance personnel, hospital administrators and the consuming public made on-site visits of almost 80% of the state's hospitals to assure the validity of the survey. The criteria used were advocated by the American Medical Association and the American Hospital Association, but to pacify the hospitals, the reference to the phrase "basic" was removed and "community" was used. The 1976 survey was conducted by mail. One can vaguely describe the difference between a general and community hospital in the availability of personnel in the emergency department, while the difference between an area and general hospital is the availability of inhouse specialty services. In Wisconsin, the specialists required to be available within the hospital were an anesthesiologist, a general surgeon, neurosurgeon, cardiothoracic surgeon, pediatrician and cardiologist. Seventy-two percent of Wisconsin's hospitals were classified as community, 25% were thought to have general capability, while 3% or four hospitals had area capability. Two of the area hospitals had medical school affiliation.

The emergency medical health care team is composed of many members who function at different times and places. The development and formation of this team took several decades and was in response to needs initiated by changes in education and emergency care. Prior to the 1940s, there was solo practice. To be responsive to the increase in scientific research and publications, specialization flourished and group practices developed to improve physician coverage. The dawn of EMS and the realization that the objective of emergency care was the provision of services and service capability caused the need and the impetus for the team approach with each member providing a link to the chain of care.

In the context of this discussion, hospital capability makes reference to a sufficient number of personnel who have had appropriate training to use available, necessary and sophisticated equipment to provide a needed service. The common denominator of all hospitals is their ability to provide stabilizing care and varying abilities to provide temporizing or definitive care. The primary objective of all hospitals must be to provide a life-saving measure for any acute medical, surgical or traumatic emergency. Many of these problems may be given additional and/or definitive care and the patient subsequently discharged. Certain cases, by virtue of the emergency or its complication, require stabilizing maneuvers at the completion of which the question must be asked, "What is the availability of definitive diagnostic and therapeutic measures?" If they are not within the hospital's capability, the patient and the problem must be transferred to another institution which has that service.

Emergency governments in many medical communities have been spending endless hours and countless dollars in trying to identify and develop some type of disaster plan. This plan is primarily directed toward nuclear bomb attacks and all other types of natural calamities. For most communities and most hospitals, a two-car accident involving multiple injuries represents a disaster, and all physicians have been party to the occasion in which they have had multiple patients enter with multiple organ system involvement, requiring multiple physician specialty or specialty service. It is for these instances that one must develop some type of a relationship in the rural community with the urban community because it is in the urban community where the specialty services are to be found.

To assure himself, his patient and the community that emergency care in all its facets is available, the physician must make a commitment. This commitment may be to relieve one's self of all the responsibility or to accept it. The motivation for making the positive commitment may originate in the prehospital, emergency department or inhospital services and, on occasion, even in hospital administration. Regardless of where the motivation for the commitment for EMS begins, it needs physician acceptance and involvement. After the commitment has been made, the hospital and its staff must survey its own resources as well as those in the area, region and state to identify the service capabilities and to become aware of its own deficiencies. This survey should relate to manpower, training, communications, equipment, vehicles and facilities. The final effort is to implement the program so that the necessary emergency services are either readily available in the hospital, its surrounding community or made available through the transfer of the patient.

Jackson County is one of the more rural counties in Wisconsin and has a population of 15,000 with its county seat being in a community of 3500. There is one hospital for the county, two nursing homes and a group practice consisting of eight physicians. In view of the fact that there are many activities, both social and otherwise, that are carried out in all four seasons and the potential for emergencies occurring at all levels, an EMS program was developed directing itself to improving the pre-hospital and the emergency department care. A trailer was converted into a mobile first aid station and used on occasions where a large number of people congregated, such as snowmobile derbies and state fairs. The station is manned by EMTs and nurses who provide the most basic of first aid. In the event treatment is needed, the patient is referred. Since the county contained 50,000 acres of forest land, winter sports were common, so a rescue sled was purchased along with a snowmobile for easy access to the ill and injured. The community's station wagons were removed, and KKK standard vehicles were obtained. In the event that an interhospital transfer of a critically ill patient was necessary, a critical care nurse with appropriate equipment was sent with the patient along with standing orders which would cover most of the situations she would be expected to encounter.

First responder training (Crash Injury Management Course) was given to the smaller community volunteer fire departments, while the main ambulance unit received EMT training. Continuing training on a semi-annual basis is available through the American Trauma Society's EMS Continuing Training Program and is provided regionally. Local continuing training efforts are provided by the physician on a monthly basis, utilizing an ED/EMT Care Critique, also developed by the American Trauma Society. These 30-minute didactic sessions, complete with case presentations, are monitored by the local physician.

The ultimate relationship between the urban and rural communities represents a push-pull mechanism which pivots on the words "need" and "services." The rural area must identify the need and the urban area responds to it. This need may be patient-orientated, and the only way the need can be responded to is by transferring the patient. The referring physician must select the most appropriate urban service and be assured that the transfer is made expeditiously and efficiently. The urban area responds by providing ready access to that service, and after the patient has been cared for, it responds by returning the patient. Urban facilities want a call made by rural physicians to make them aware of the case and are desirous of a transfer form with all of the pertinent information. If the rural area is made to make the call and forwards the information to the urban area, they deserve a call back, stating that the transfer was made safely and a report given on the primary assessment. A formal summary and follow-up report should precede the patient's return home.

The rural need may be related to manpower, the training for that manpower, the equipment that they would use, or it may be in transportation capability or specialty services. The urban area should respond to these needs by assisting in providing training and making available mobile specialty care vehicles.

Self-Evaluation Quiz

1. Categorization guidelines used by states in identifying hospital capabilities are uniform.
   a) True
   b) False
2. Only specialty hospitals should be able to provide life-saving measures.
   a) True
   b) False
3. All hospitals and medical staffs can provide equal service.
   a) True
   b) False
4. The motivation to improve emergency medical care delivery must begin with the physician.
   a) True
   b) False
5. The primary purpose for surveying the community's emergency medical care resources is to identify deficiencies and emergency care capability.
   a) True
   b) False

Answers on page 289.

Observations on the Urban Aspects of an EMS System

Alan Dimick, M.D.

Objectives

Rural/urban relationships in the provision of medical care continue to be a major challenge, because these two areas are so disparate in their natural concerns and points of view. This discussion will center on the unique factors in both rural and urban settings, and in particular will address emergency medical care provided in each. Methods to utilize the best portions of both rural and urban emergency medical care will be detailed, as well as how they should be coordinated to provide the best possible care to the patient with a medical emergency.

The urban tertiary care facilities and personnel have much to offer to their counterparts in the rural areas, primarily for consultation and referral of patients requiring higher levels of care. There is a definite need to maintain excellent working relationships and communication between both areas. Those in the urban setting must keep in mind the circumstances regarding medical facilities and trained personnel in rural areas are not as complete and diversified as in urban settings. This is a dynamic relationship which those in the urban setting must continually cultivate and improve. The interaction and communication between rural and urban needs to be nurtured and improved in both directions. We must do this for the benefit of our patients.

I might illustrate this by telling you about one way in which Alabama has done this. We utilize a WATS line, called MIST

Alan Dimick, M.D., Associate Professor of Surgery, University of Alabama Medical Center, Birmingham; Member, Board of Directors, American Trauma Society.

(Medical Information Service Via Telephone) for any physician in the state to be able to call a specialist at the University of Alabama Medical Center in Birmingham about any problem he has. In other words, he can get almost immediate consultation by calling a toll-free telephone number which is answered at our University Hospital. MIST actually started when our Dean of Medicine was in private practice previously in Selma, Alabama, about seven years ago. He said there were many times he wished he had the ability to call someone for a consultation on a moment's notice.

When he became Dean of the Medical School, he implemented this concept, so that now the rural physician can call us to consult on his problem, which we may be able to handle over the telephone, or he can transfer his patient to us. Obviously, it is the decision of the rural physician as to what he wants to do with his patient.

This does several things. It makes the specialist in the medical center more aware of the problems out in the community hospitals and physicians' offices in the state and provides a type of continuing education as to what the current therapy for a particular disorder or illness may be. Then the specialist at our medical center can send the rural physician reprints, a bibliography or other information on this particular problem.

This has worked so well that the Alabama legislature has funded this as part of the budget of the UAB Medical Center for the past five years. It works very well not only for physicians, but also for nurses, dietitians and other health workers who may have a problem requiring consultation.

Obviously, it is ideal for the emergency situation, because at any hour of the day or night the physician in a small community can contact a specialist in any area of medicine by simply dialing a toll-free telephone number. We have feedback from the physicians in the rural areas that they really enjoy this ability to talk to a specialist in the medical center and usually can get a consultation within five minutes after they call.

There is a special type of transportation which they have developed in Wisconsin and elsewhere. A team of physicians, nurses and technicians retrieve a patient at a local hospital who may be unstable. The team then stabilizes the patient at the referring hospital and brings the patient back into the tertiary care center in a mobile intensive care unit. This does not happen all the time, but it can occur in certain areas where you want to be certain that the patient has safe transportation to the tertiary care center. A number of states are now doing this for their tertiary transportation. This obviously does not replace primary transportation by ambulance. This transfer to the tertiary care center is accomplished with a complete team to stabilize the patient and continue the care for his multiple problems.

Transfer agreements should be initiated by the referring hospitals in the rural communities and then be sent to the receiving hospital for signature, because this is the way the patients flow. The transfer agreement works at both ends. It makes the physician referring the patient consider what needs to be done and to whom he needs to talk. At the other end of the transfer agreement is the receiving physician, who should send back information to the referring physician both acutely after the patient arrives or later at the time of discharge from the medical center. This makes the specialist in the receiving hospital know that he must let the referring physician know what has happened to his patient. Information must go in both directions in order to have optimum patient care.

Many names are assigned to tertiary transfer vehicles. In Columbia, South Carolina, they have a neonatal transfer unit, which is a modified mobile home, and they call it "the stork." I thought that was an appropriate name for a bus that goes out and picks up critically ill neonates. And then they corrected me, they said, "No, that stands for Speedy Transfer of Risky Kids (STORK)."

They have recently changed the term from just high-risk neonates to perinatal medicine, which emphasizes they take care of the mother and the child before birth, when they can identify the high-risk problem in pregnancy.

The Federal Aviation Administration tried earlier this year to establish standards for air ambulances, but were unsuccessful because of the strong opposition from people in the flying ambulance business. Much to my distress it was mostly physicians who were involved in the business for profit of flying ambulances. Currently the air ambulances operating do not provide anything close to what a ground ambulance should provide. For instance, quite often they do not even provide oxygen or heat in the compartment. You probably read some stories in the *Parade Magazine* earlier this year about the sorry state of air ambulances throughout the nation. Currently there are no regulations concerning air ambulances, but there certainly need to be. A few states have established regulations. I think Arizona and Tennessee have some fairly good standards. Nationally, I do not think there is enough standardization of it. I am concerned because I am in charge of the burn unit at the University of Alabama in Birmingham, and some of my patients have had to be transferred by air. The private air ambulances that have been contracted to transfer my patients are atrocious. If they were ground ambulances they would be "grounded."

Self-Evaluation Quiz

1. Transfer agreements should be initiated by the referring hospital in rural communities.
   a) True
   b) False
2. It is not necessary for the receiving physician to have further contact with the referring physician.
   a) True
   b) False
3. Air ambulances provide excellent care comparable to ground ambulances.
   a) True
   b) False
4. MIST is an instrument for respiration.
   a) True
   b) False

Answers on page 289.

Preparation for the Emergency

Mildred Fincke, R.N.

Objectives

1. To gain insight into the role of the emergency department and the entire hospital in meeting the open-ended emergency situation of serving or arranging for service to all of the injured under any circumstances.
2. To appreciate the value of *preparation* and *planning* in emergency service.

In this presentation I shall speak of the preparations in the emergency department which are essential for care of emergency patients. It is well recognized that patients are still being lost unnecessarily because of system failures. The hospital emergency department is the crucial entry point into the health care system for patients. How, then, does the preparation for the emergency begin, and what is the plan for emergency care in your own hospital?

The communications system is one of the most important factors and the backbone of the emergency medical services (EMS) system. A good communications network provides for the coordination of the many agencies and personnel which become involved in the emergency care of either a single injured patient or mass casualties. Centralized communication and dispatch are crucial to a good EMS system.

There has been dramatic improvement in access of the public to emergency care, quality of care at the scene and in transit, and the readiness of emergency departments to provide adequate care. Good effective care to the victim for transport from the scene of accident to the hospital is vital to effective

---

Mildred Fincke, R.N., Administrative Director, Emergency/Ambulatory Services, Allegheny General Hospital, Pittsburgh, Pa.

medical care. Outcome data in areas that have been studied show a positive impact of the EMS on morbidity and mortality.

The communications network sets the pace for hospital emergency departments to go on alert for the transfer of the patient and to set up and be prepared for the emergency trauma. In many parts of the country, hospital-to-hospital and hospital-to-ambulance voice linkage is combined with telemetry of biomedical data. This allows for continuous monitoring of the patient during transportation and for verbal orders to trained ambulatory personnel, such as starting intravenous therapy, administering drugs and defibrillating. Medical command responsibility either at a hospital or at a community-based central emergency communication center is essential. Every physician giving command and the EMT receiving the command must be aware of the qualifications of those giving patient care. The key word is trust.

The general rule of law adopted by the courts has been that a hospital which operates an emergency department as a service to the public and holds out such service to the public is required to accept patients who present themselves for care, treat them without negligence and arrange for a referral if the hospital does not have the necessary facilities or capabilities for that patient's care. Hopefully, this is what will be called categorization, or development of a system that provides for facilities assessment of patient classification.

Many emergency departments still lack a good organizational structure and an adequate emergency plan of action. To provide a foundation for an effective emergency department, each hospital must evaluate its capabilities and then devise its operational plan. What might be good in Pittsburgh may not be good in Atlanta or in other parts of the country. The same is true of staffing patterns. The degree of organization and readiness in the emergency area is vital in the successful management of injured patients. Trained physicians, nurses and ancillary persons must be immediately available. The triage and patient flow process keeps the emergency department on an alert basis at all times. Also, there must be treatment rooms ready and properly equipped. Since quick decisions must be made by the emergency nurse, it is essential that equipment be listed and checked for adequacies and readiness for use.

Protocols and procedures must be written for the department and the staff knowledgeable of their purpose. Standing orders are a must and evaluation of patient care by audit is essential for efficient operation. Critiques of pre-hospital patient care and of the emergency department for management of specific cases provide an evaluation of the way the EMS system works.

It is most important to find out if the pre-hospital care has been adequate and whether the emergency department has been alerted to the patient who is coming in, has made proper preparation and whether the plan of care was adequate. Regardless of the hospital's capabilities, you must know what preparations you have made for the care of the injured in your emergency setting. Whether you are a large metropolitan urban area, community or rural hospital, you are held accountable for the care you give and the preparation it takes to give that care.

The seven standards promulgated by the Joint Commission on Accreditation of Hospitals (JCAH) on emergency services provide the guidelines to preparation for emergency services. The Joint Commission formerly had five standards — about two pages of printing. There are now seven standards and these comprise almost a complete document. If you follow the seven standards you will be meeting the requirements on the establishment of emergency services for accreditation.

As emergency nurses, you cannot be haphazard in your management of emergency patients. There are many hospital emergency departments that cannot accommodate or cope with the magnitude of trauma injuries. What is the standard and the expectation of emergency care at your hospital? There must be well-trained personnel in the emergency department to provide an efficient emergency system. There must be nurses who can be responsible for nursing activities that will preserve life and function and who can expertly provide a nursing assessment of the patient's injuries.

Also important is a systematic assessment of the patient's injuries to determine the urgency of treatment and to prevent an oversight on any concealed injuries. Top priority is given to evaluating and managing life-threatening situations. Priorities of care for trauma patients in order of urgency are as follows: airway problems, hemorrhage, shock, open wounds and closed fractures.

Preparation for any emergency — whatever your own emergency department's capabilities may be — starts with a responsible nurse in charge, since well-run emergency departments must be staffed by properly trained personnel. Orientation and education of the nurses and the nursing staff are vital to a well-organized emergency department. Therefore, continuing education is essential. Assessment, evaluation and reevaluation must be an ongoing process.

Statistical data-gathering from trip sheets, radio communication, emergency department records and outcome audits assist one in the triage system of making things happen. The emergency nurse is the backbone of the emergency department, just as the communications system is the backbone of the EMS. The nurse sets the pace, but the process of care can be carried out properly only with a good ongoing physician-nurse-administration relationship. Documentation for the pre-hospital-to-hospital process is vital to the care of the patient. Trip sheets must be a part of your emergency department record. They are used not only for your information in the emergency department, but also by physicians and nurses on the floor when the patient is admitted. These physicians and nurses want to know what happened to the patient before he arrived at the emergency department, what happened in the emergency department and, then, what will happen when the patient reaches the floor.

Morbidity and mortality records on a 24-hour basis should be part of your emergency system, so that you have answers to these questions: Did we do the right thing for that particular patient in the emergency department? Did the patient die within 24 hours? How many patients came into the emergency department and died within 24 hours after admission? This kind of statistical-gathering is important.

Standing orders to initiate care with or without physicians are a must. Many hospitals do not have standing orders and, as a result, there is utter chaos in the emergency department because no one knows who is going to do what, when it will be done and how it is to be done. Such situations do occur everywhere in the country. You can walk into many area hospitals throughout the United States and be told their emergency departments are well organized, but when you ask to see their standing orders, procedure and policy books, and process and outcome audits you are told they are still working on them. They have probably been working on them for many years and never finished the product, or if they did during those many years, they failed to keep the records updated.

Protocols and procedures must be written and approved by the triage system. This means that the physician, the administration and nursing must know what is in the hospital procedure and protocol book. They must approve your standing orders. After all, there is a medicolegal issue in the emergency department. You will prevent problems many times by having well-documented records, and well-documented records follow from well-designed protocols and procedures.

You must also know your community resources. What are the capabilities of other local area hospitals? Do you have transfer agreements between your hospital and another hospital? What happens when a call comes in from some of the areas across the country, bringing you a severely burned patient because there is not a burn center within that area? What is the transfer protocol from your hospital to a burn center hospital? Do you send a patient who is not stabilized or send him out without proper stabilization? This does happen. We are a 726-bed acute care hospital, with a hospital-based helicopter system which recently went into active operation. We find that patients to be transported have not been stabilized at the transferring hospital before the flight team arrives.

There must be advanced routines for disaster preparedness. It is easy to take care of just one patient when you get the command that there is one patient coming into your emergency department with multiple trauma. You simply go into action. But what happens if there are 5, 10, 15, 20 or 25 such patients? Do you know the department's capabilities? Do you call the hospitals around you every day on your radio communication system to find out what their bed situation is and whether their emergency department is overflowing with patients waiting for beds? This is all part of being prepared for any disaster or any emergency.

Job descriptions are essential. Do you know what your employees can and cannot do? Do you have a list in your hospital that tells you what is and is not permitted for treatment in your emergency department?

The Joint Commission on Accreditation of Hospitals recently visited our hospital. We were not perfect for no one is perfect. The JCAH reviewers went through all of the seven JCAH standards and justification was requested for every positive statement we made. They did not accept our assurances that we complied with the standards; they asked to see and inspect.

Transfer agreements between hospitals are very important. It is not only a question of the legal issue of who is responsible for the patient from your hospital to where he is going, but you must be certain you have stabilized the patient adequately and properly documented the entire procedure.

Be certain of protocols for admitted patients and the means of following through on patient care after the emergency. You may find that you are having multiple trauma victims coming into the emergency department when you are already overflowing with patients. You have patients there waiting for beds because there are no beds available in the house. Then you hear that you will receive five or ten more patients. Do you have a plan of action as to how you are going to handle them?

Advance notice of impending arrivals in the emergency department with good data information is very essential. It is easy to say be on the alert, but what do you know about the patient? Do you have a good dispatch system? Does your dispatcher or your medical command physician report to your emergency department on what is coming in? In-depth detail is not necessary, but pertinent information is because it sets the pace for the emergency department. If you know the patient has fractures, you know exactly what you are going to have to do. You know what equipment should be ready immediately and what your plan of care will be.

Your plan of action is merely alerting your staff by assessing the data given by the medical dispatcher. This sounds simple, but much effort goes into preplanning for the emergency department. All the ground rules are laid down, as mentioned earlier — the standing orders, etc. But what about your staff? Are they attuned to what is going on when the patient arrives? Or do you fear that word "turf?" Are you afraid that if everyone knows what is going on there will be utter chaos? Do you have a plan that puts all of your staff where they should be? Are your triage system and your patient flow patterns working? Is your triage nurse in position? I am assuming that you use a triage system — whether you are a small or a large hospital. Someone must be the triage person — a nurse or an ombudsman out front who is talking to the patients and their families. This triage person will eliminate many complaints which might otherwise go to administration and, also, will prevent patient flow from backing up.

Orientation and reorientation are needed not only for your emergency staff, but also for your community. Does your triage nurse do any educating of the patients in the waiting room? Does she keep them informed on what to expect? Does she tell them that there may be long delays and explain why? Are these patients alerted to the fact that casualties are coming in? Is your triage nurse able to move them out of your emergency department into an ambulatory care setting? What are the standing rules for your triage nurse to follow? Who is the boss? Do you have a good physician working with you who is backing you up all the way? This last factor is most important.

Rosters for physician coverage should always be updated, current and in front of you so that you know who is on call and where each one can be reached. There is nothing more embarrassing — and sometimes critical — than failure to find a physician who has told you he is on call that night, will return later or let you know where he is and then failed to inform you of his whereabouts. It can and does happen. Who is the responsible person who tells the physician that he cannot go out because he is on call and supposed to be in the hospital for 24 hours that day? How strong are you in your emergency department? Do you have the support of the administration, physicians and nurses all saying the same thing at the same time and who are in agreement on all policies and procedures?

Preparing for the emergency perhaps begins with a call from the EMT. You assess what he has told you and then go into action. Do you notify the x-ray department right away? Are you supposed to notify the laboratory immediately that the patient is arriving? Perhaps it is 5:00 o'clock in the evening and everything except the emergency department closes at 5:00 p.m. Suppose you are called at 4:30 p.m. Do you call the laboratory and the x-ray department and tell them you have a patient arriving and that you do not know whether their services will be needed, but request they stand by until the patient comes in? This is all preplanning. Do you call the blood bank, inhalation therapy, the operating room? What about your nursing service? Do you notify nursing service? Suppose it is 5:00 p.m. and the director of inpatient nursing has left for the day. Do you alert her to casualties arriving so that she can check the bed situation for you? Are there enough nurses in the house? Do you have a 24-hour backup in your operating room? Do these nurses stay in the hospital or are they within 20 minutes from the hospital?

All of this must be written and documented so that every new nurse coming into your department will follow the same procedures. There can be no "ifs, ands or buts." You are responsible for the system that makes the emergency department function effectively and efficiently. Breakdowns in the system do occur, but what do you do about them? There can be times when you have alerted the x-ray department, the laboratory, the operating room, the admitting office for bed availability and suddenly you find out that what you may need for the patient is not readily available. Who is your backup and who does the coordinating to see that the "whole team is working together"? There must be a system worked out. This is important to avoid accusations that the department is shirking the job or evading its responsibilities. The team working together makes good patient care happen.

If you are already overbooked with patients, admissions are most frustrating. You have patients waiting for beds and suddenly the EMTs call and say they are bringing in two additional patients. What do you do in that situation? Sometimes I look at the emergency department and I think it is the most chaotic, disorganized *organized* system in the hospital. However, patients and professional staff not connected with the emergency department sometimes consider it quite disorganized. They do not realize that emergency nurses and physicians are attuned to that department, know very well its procedures and protocols and the way it functions, and all of them have everything in their heads, organized and tabulated. They know the plan of action they will take under given circumstances and possible contingencies, and they are ready when the patient arrives.

Consider equipment. What kind of equipment do you have? Since nurses and other personnel in the emergency department are required to make quick and accurate medical decisions, equipment and supplies must be adequate and in the unit. None of the equipment in the emergency department should ever be borrowed or removed from the premises because no one can foresee when or how quickly it may be needed. The lack of any necessary equipment could easily cost the patient his life and result in a legal entanglement for the hospital and the responsible medical and nursing staff.

All personnel working in the emergency department must know the location of every piece of equipment. There should be a list posted of all supplies and equipment with the quotas of these items noted. This may sound trivial, but it is a *must*. You should be checking and rechecking your rooms, and everyone should know exactly what is in every room and where the essential trays, tubes, splints and medications are located.

All nurses and medical personnel must be trained to use every item of the intricate, sophisticated electrical and electronic monitoring equipment in the department. There can be no excuse for not knowing how to use it or for not knowing whether it has been checked, how often it is checked and when it was last rechecked. Do you also do this in your drug room? Do you know when the pharmacy department last checked the drug room? Do you know when the nursing staff responsible for this assignment last checked it?

All emergency supplies must be clearly marked and strategically placed. Equipment and supplies must be constantly checked, both for adequacy and readiness and for maintenance care. Cardiac and pulmonary resuscitation equipment must be located conveniently on a resuscitation cart which is movable easily from one area of the emergency department to another.

Communications equipment is a necessity in the emergency department as well as in any other department of the hospital. Direct telephone linkage to other in-hospital facilities, such as the laboratory, x-ray department, operating room, pharmacy and admission office lends immeasurable efficiency to the emergency department. No emergency department can afford delays in this system. Five years ago we moved into a new emergency department. We are now renovating the department again to provide for its own x-ray room and to improve the communications system. Direct telephone lines to crucial services will be provided. A busy emergency nurse does not have time to wait on the telephone for a free line. The clerk who could do this may also be busy or she may not be on duty. Thus, hospital communication to vital services by direct link is the most efficient and effective way to operate.

Interdepartment services must be immediately accessible and available. If they are not, the efficiency of the emergency department suffers and the patient can be seriously and adversely affected. For example, the delay in obtaining an available operating room and in initiating x-ray and diagnostic laboratory studies or in obtaining the services of the blood bank can bring about problems which, in addition to influencing patient care, may give rise to medicolegal issues.

We come to a final factor directly and importantly related to the emergency department — your disaster plan. What is your pre-hospital emergency disaster plan and do you know how well and smoothly it works? There should be two simulated disaster runs per year to keep the emergency department staff and hospital personnel alert. The coordinator of the plan should be the physician in the emergency department with the nursing team. How many of you work in a hospital where the disaster plan is formulated by individuals other than personnel from the emergency department? This is totally unacceptable.

In summary, since it is inclusive of many medical and nursing disciplines, emergency medicine is dependent upon these disciplines for back-up support if optimal care is to be given. The practice of emergency medicine is best carried out by the physicians and nurses with a special interest and expertise in this field of care, trained in emergency medicine and, therefore, best qualified to assess the medical problems presented and deal with them completely and expeditiously. The roles of the emergency physician and the emergency nurse are essentially episodic and must include the capability to initiate resuscitative and life-support measures with a wide spectrum of mechanical and electronic devices. Extrahospital, interdepartmental and intradepartmental communications input from your medical staff and house physicians and the proper use of your facilities and equipment are all important and helpful in the delivery of emergency medicine. Ultimately, decisions for the organization and the function of the emergency department are within the province of the emergency department committee. Do you have such a committee in your hospital and who is responsible for your emergency department? Is your emergency committee composed of physicians who are not even part of the emergency system? Day-to-day operations and decisions must be made by the emergency physician and the emergency nurse with input from all of the emergency department personnel. Team effort is the key to a well-organized and well-administered department toward achieving its primary objective of giving each emergency patient the best obtainable level of care and of assuring prompt, adequate examination and treatment for all patients who require care in the emergency department.

Self-Evaluation Quiz

1. The backbone of the EMS system is the:
   a) Head nurse
   b) Radiology department
   c) Communications system
   d) Triage committee
2. Voice linkage systems:
   a) Are not permitted by state law to provide telemetry of biomedical data
   b) May telemeter biomedical data if the physician is in the ambulance
   c) Include telemetry of biomedical data in some parts of the country
3. Verbal orders to trained ambulatory personnel include defibrillating, IV therapy and administering drugs.
   a) True
   b) False
4. At the present time:
   a) No rule of law has been applied by courts to EMS
   b) A general rule of law has been adopted for hospitals that offer service to the public
   c) The courts have forbade the hospitals to offer care to the injured on the streets
   d) None of the above

5. Protocols and procedures:
   a) Are anathema to a good, flexible EMS system
   b) Tend to discourage initiative in real emergencies
   c) Are essential for EMS
   d) Are permitted if the physician-in-charge allows sidestepping them when they hamper speed and virtuosity
6. The Joint Commission on Accreditation of Hospitals (JCAH) promulgated ______ standards.
   a) 2
   b) 4
   c) 7
   d) 8
7. Airway problems have first priority in emergency care.
   a) True
   b) False
8. Trip sheets are not a part of the emergency department record.
   a) True
   b) False
9. The author suggests two simulated disaster runs per year to keep emergency department staff and hospital personnel alert.
   a) True
   b) False

Answers on page 289.

Panel Discussion: ED/EMT Care Critiques

Moderator: Charles Aprahamian, M.D.
Panelists: Dottie South, R.N.
Steve Asbury, REMT

Moderator: When the American Trauma Society conducted a survey of hospitals to determine their involvement in ambulance personnel/emergency department personnel critiques, it was noted that approximately one third of the hospitals were conducting these conferences, and in those, approximately 40% were held monthly. The American Trauma Society/Wisconsin Division recognized the need for these programs and has been developing what is termed an ED/EMT Care Critique. At these critiques, didactic information is presented and followed with case presentations which usually deal with the subject discussed. It is believed these critiques are important because of the platoon system of care now practiced. In the past, there was just one member of the team — the inhouse physician. It has always been amazing to hear of the medical community being so concerned with the patient once he arrived at the hospital but having little concern over what happened to the patient in the pre-hospital setting or even after he has been seen in the emergency room. But once the physician was called to see the patient, he would exclaim, "My God, we are going to mobilize all the resources that are available to help this patient." Over a period of time and due to the impetus of EMS, it has been noted that our priorities are

Charles Aprahamian, M.D., Assistant Professor of Surgery, Medical College of Wisconsin, Milwaukee; Dottie South, R.N., Manager, Emergency Room, Brookwood Hospital, Homewood, Ala.; and Steve Asbury, REMT, EMS Coordinator, Pee Dee Regional Health Systems Agency, Florence, S.C.

changing; the main objective in emergency care is to provide services or the availability of services. As a consequence, the team has enlarged. We now have a first platoon which represents the first responder and ambulance personnel. The second platoon is the emergency department with its nurse and physician. The third platoon remains the inhouse physicians and nurses.

The process of emergency health care delivery begins with the initial assessment which represents an itemization of all of the patient's presenting problems. The triage is to give priority to the problems that were itemized, thereby selecting the most urgent problem first. The third step in emergency care delivery consists in providing the life-saving care for that priority illness or injury followed by the initiation of other life support measures. This sequence of assessment, triage, provision of emergency care and initiation of life support must be periodically reviewed to assure that the process is smooth and appropriate. The ED/EMT Care Critique is one means of auditing that process.

The first case for review is an automobile accident in which four people are involved. The first patient is a 56-year-old man who, following the accident, noted the onset of severe chest pain. He subsequently became diaphoretic and preferred to sit rather than lie down. Someone at the scene noted rattling in the victim's chest. The second victim is an 18-year-old male who was thrown against the windshield and sustained facial injuries as well as a deformed elbow. The third victim is a man in his forties. He was intoxicated or at least his breath had the distinctive odor of alcohol. In addition, he was semistuporous and had an avulsion laceration of the scalp. The fourth victim is an unconscious male. Someone noted that his pulse was thready, and they thought he might be hypotensive.

These are the four cases. Now, we will ask our pre-hospital platoon — the ambulance crew who was there at the scene — What did you see? What did you do? What are some of your thoughts?

Mr. Asbury: I shall describe the accident in a little more detail. This accident occurred at 1:15 a.m. on a Sunday; outdoor temperature was in the mid-50s. We received a telephone call for a motor vehicle accident, and while en route, we received word via radio that there had been a single car accident and that the police were already on the scene. There were four critically injured patients, and they thought one was already dead. The dispatcher advised that he was dispatching a second ambulance as well as the fire department rescue team. While en route, my partner and I discussed the potentiality of this type of accident and we each decided to take two patients initially. When we arrived at the scene, the police were already there, and the fire department rescue team arrived within seconds.

The man suffering chest pains was seated on the curb and was being assisted by the police officer. We bypassed him and went first to the unconscious victim. I did an assessment of his airway, breathing and pulse and determined that this patient was in need of rapid transportation and initial care. We did some suctioning to his upper airways, a cervical collar was placed and we moved him to a spine board.

Simultaneously, the other EMT went to assist the two other patients. The one with facial injuries and deformed elbow was found seated in the right front seat of the car. The EMT checked for airway patency and noted that the grossly deformed elbow did not have a distal radial pulse and the arm was somewhat cool. The other patient did smell strongly of alcohol. His airway was adequate, his pulse was strong and his rate was adequate.

The unconscious patient who was placed on a spine board with a cervical collar was moved to the ambulance. His airway was monitored and his pharynx was suctioned periodically. The patient with facial injuries was also placed in the ambulance. Care was directed toward his airway. The arm was splinted in the position in which it was found.

The patient with chest pain was placed on a primary cot with oxygen by mask, running at 8 liters/min. The intoxicated patient had his wounds bandaged, a cervical collar was placed, and he was strapped to a backboard and put on the squad bench. Each ambulance established contact with the hospital. The hospital-based physician wanted the chest patient placed in a semi-seated position with an IV of D-5-W started. An EKG strip was transmitted. After review, the physician ordered morphine and Lasix. The intoxicated patient with the facial laceration received an IV of Ringer's lactate.

The ambulance with the unconscious patient received orders for airway maintenance as aggressively as needed to assure a patent airway. We were encouraged to call back to the hospital if we thought there was a need for an esophageal airway. An IV of Ringer's lactate was started, and we were instructed to run it wide open. Because of the continued low vital signs, we received an order to use the MAST suit. Regarding the patient with the facial injuries and deformed elbow, we were given instructions to continue to monitor airway, start an IV of Ringer's lactate, to keep open and transport as quickly as possible because of the potential nerve and/or vascular damage associated with the elbow injury.

The ambulances arrived at the hospital approximately 20 minutes after leaving the scene. The elapsed time from accident to arrival at the hospital was approximately 50 minutes. It took the EMTs and paramedics approximately 20 to 25 minutes at the scene to treat, stabilize and begin the transfer of the patient.

Moderator: Mr. Asbury, did both of the vehicles go to the same hospital?

Mr. Asbury: Yes, that is correct.

Moderator: Is there only one hospital in town?

Mr. Asbury: It was the only one at that time which could receive four patients because they had a physician on call in the hospital.

Moderator: That is interesting. I just wonder how many hospitals have the capability of caring for four different patients with four different organ systems, requiring four different types of specialty services. But if that is what you have available in your community, that's what you must use.

Now let us ask our emergency department personnel some questions. When the first ambulance comes in, you note you have an unconscious individual who apparently has head injuries and is also hypotensive. He has been treated en route with fluids and MAST suit. I am going to change some of the circumstances of this case to make you the only person there. It just so happens that the physician who was on call is just not available. His phone is out of order and he is not likely to be there for the next 15 minutes. You will have the primary responsibility for assessing and caring for this patient and your concern should be directed to the first vehicle which has the unconscious patient and the victim with facial injuries and a deformed elbow.

Ms. South: Naturally, it is a typical day in the emergency room, or a typical early morning in the emergency room. The ER physician is inhouse answering a code. I would rather think it was that than a telephone out of order. In the head injury victim, the airway management is most important. The IV has already been started. We transfer the patient off of the backboard onto an immobilizer while still maintaining the splinting of the back. The patient does have a cervical collar, but it is important to immobilize the neck with sand bags.

I listen to the EMT regarding his assessment of the patient to determine what has transpired. Even though we have had voice communications, he can now give me additional information. Laboratory is ready, and we draw CBC, blood sugar, blood gases and electrolytes. Extra blood is drawn in the event additional tests are deemed necessary after the x-rays have been taken. As far as x-rays are concerned, we will get the routine cervical spines, cross-table laterals of the neck, skull films, facial bones, etc. I am allowed to do this because of standing orders which are the result of the protocols developed in our department. While it may not be standard in other hospitals, in many of the unconscious patients brought to our department, we do give a bolus of 50% glucose with the consideration that some of the patients are hypoglycemic.

Regarding the patient with facial injuries and deformed elbow, we check the splints, put the arm on pillows and place ice on the swollen area. Appropriate x-rays of the face, skull, cervical spine and the elbow are taken.

Moderator: The unconscious patient who has a weak, thready pulse and hypotension does have evidence of bilateral periorbital ecchymosis or the "raccoon eyes." What do you think of that?

Ms. South: Before I answer that, I want to ask Mr. Asbury if this is the patient he put a MAST suit on. I question application of a MAST suit in head injury cases.

Moderator: Does anyone else question application of the MAST suit in head injury cases?

Response from floor: Not only do I question the use of the MAST suit, but I question the order for a large volume IV fluid.

Moderator: Perhaps I should respond to these concerns. If I saw that patient, I would say that he probably has a basilar skull fracture. In fact, I would consider an anterior basilar skull fracture because, with anterior basilar skull fractures, one develops the "raccoon eyes." If it were a posterior basilar skull fracture, patients often get ecchymosis about the mastoid process which is called Battle's sign. There is one other thing I look for in head injuries and that is the "halo sign." Halo sign is a red center with a yellow outside which indicates that the meninges have been violated and the cerebrospinal fluid and blood are mixed. As this fluid comes out of the ear or nose and drips on the sheet, the blood which has a greater molecular weight diffuses slowly and stays in the center while the cerebrospinal fluid diffuses more rapidly, giving a yellow halo about the red center. A halo sign signifies to me that the patient has a serious head injury.

I have never seen a head injury admitted with hypotension with the hypotension being caused by the head injury. If you have a head injury plus hypotension or other evidence of shock, the patient has an injury elsewhere, and that injury elsewhere is either in his chest, abdomen or his extremities, be it soft tissue injury or multiple fractures with blood loss. We instruct our EMTs and nurses that if you have a head injury associated with hypotension, the MAST suit is appropriate because you are using it to increase venous return to the heart.

Mr. Asbury: We were taught that if the patient has a head injury and is hypotensive, we treat the hypotension and let the physician worry about the head injury. We also provide airway management and use the esophageal airway. We always put cervical collars on these patients.

Ms. South: The person in the audience questioned the large bore needle. This is a lifeline, and even if it is just a head injury or associated injuries, you can always restart it in a smaller vein, but if you get total collapse, then, of course, you appreciate your large bore needle.

Response from floor: I would question the idea of having given 50 cc of 50% glucose to the unconscious patient with the idea that he may be in insulin shock when the likelihood is that he is suffering from trauma and not insulin shock.

Moderator: I cannot see where 50 cc of 50% glucose is going to do much harm and it is possible that it may do some good. In any event, if it is part of a protocol, one should follow it.

Response from floor: In regard to that issue, it has always been my understanding that you really do not know what happened prior to head injury and it may be that the patient collapsed and secondarily suffered the head injury. So giving him the 50% dextrose is not going to hurt anything, and it may help.

Moderator: I should like to consider the 56-year-old man with chest pain. What was he given in the field, Mr. Asbury?

Mr. Asbury: Oxygen by mask, IV 5% dextrose in water to keep open, Lasix and morphine.

Moderator: You have now seen the patient who has chest pain, IV, oxygen, Lasix and morphine. What are you going to do?

Ms. South: This sounds like a typical cardiac patient. I am glad to know that in South Carolina they are allowed to use narcotics or carry narcotics on board. In Alabama, they are not allowed to do so. Here again, there is a difference in emergency care delivery. I question the high volume of oxygen. You did say 8 liters, didn't you?

Mr. Asbury: Yes.

Response from floor: I believe the Department of Transportation booklet entitled *Emergency Victim Care Manual* tends to recommend higher liter flow than we do in our hospital base. I know that in training our paramedics we usually gear them to lower liter flow of oxygen based on the fact that we found the maximum of 6 liters is usually adequate unless patients are in severe respiratory distress.

Moderator: In the Milwaukee Paramedic Program, we never give morphine or analgesics in the field for any medical condition, any surgical condition, other than an entrapped limb. In every other case, we do not feel that morphine is an emergency drug and we do not feel it needs to be given in the field. If they do have pain for cardiac disease, oxygen should relieve most of it. Let us say that the cardiac patient was admitted to the CCU where he has a cardiac arrest and they defibrillate him.

How about the patient with the facial injury? What happens to him? What problems would we expect to have with that type of injury?

Ms. South: This person, of course, would need a complete assessment. We would totally undress the patient and look for other injuries while we maintain his airway. Appropriate x-rays would be taken of his face, neck and elbows.

Moderator: Would anyone handle it differently?

Question from floor: No mention was made of his elbow. Would that not be a primary problem?

Moderator: No, I don't think so. If I saw the patient, my concern would be the facial injury with a midface fracture and loss of airway. I think airway would take precedence over everything else in his case. I would try and stabilize the airway in whatever way possible, choosing either a nasopharyngeal airway and, if need be, an endotracheal airway. Once that patient is stabilized, I would attend to the other two or three patients to see how they were doing. If they were not in any acute distress, then I would pay particular attention to the deformed elbow to determine if it is either dislocated and/or broken. Would anyone else respond differently?

Response from floor: On the airway management, the squad has already taken care of the airway. The patient has been without a pulse or has experienced a neurovascular deficit for probably 1½ hours by this time. I think the elbow would become very important!

Moderator: Would anyone else like to comment?

Response from floor: I agree that the elbow should be given the next priority after the airway because of the possibility of the loss of limb.

Moderator: The fourth case is the alcoholic. Can we call him an alcoholic? Should we take a blood alcohol? Do we have to? I have been doing this study in Milwaukee, and I am amazed to find the incidence of alcoholism in the acutely ill patient. Some of the pulseless nonbreathers as well as some young children come in with high alcoholic content. We have seen them with medical, surgical and traumatic problems. The level of alcohol should not be obtained just to label the individual as an alcoholic, but to assist you in making the diagnosis and caring for him afterwards. You must be able to answer the question, "Is the patient unconscious due to his alcoholic state or is this a patient with a head injury complicated with an alcoholic state?" Let us go to another case for discussion.

The next case is a 48-year-old male who suffers an industrial accident in which his distal arm is amputated. He is found by the pre-hospital personnel.

Mr. Asbury: Let me describe the scene of the accident in a little greater detail. He was working on a construction crew.

While they were stacking some beams, he received a reasonably clean amputation to the lower left arm. We noted if he had any other injuries, took a brief medical history relating to past medical and surgical problems and inquired about allergies. We found no significant past history, and there were no other associated injuries. We bandaged, mobilized and elevated the injured part. He was placed on a long spine board for the ease of movement and put into the ambulance. While I was conducting the patient survey, my partner examined the severed hand and lower arm. He noted that the amputation was clean. From the ambulance he obtained a sterile burn sheet, bandaging supplies, two plastic bags and sterile saline. He bandaged the severed ends, completely wrapping the severed part in the sterile sheet, and irrigated it with sterile saline. The part was then placed in a plastic bag and sealed. He placed the first plastic bag inside of the second and added ice. Ice is generally found at construction sites, since construction workers like to drink ice water all year round, summer or winter, and they generally carry Igloo type containers of ice. We transported the patient to the hospital with a flashing red light and sirens on. We established radio contact with the emergency room, describing the accident and the patient, and notified the base that the severed part had been properly cared for and was being transported with the patient. We wondered about the patient being a possible replantation candidate.

Moderator: Mr. Asbury, let us say that for one reason or another, somebody from the work crew had put on a tourniquet. Now what?

Mr. Asbury: We would bandage the stump, elevate it and remove the tourniquet.

Moderator: Ms. South, I am giving you the patient as delivered by Mr. Asbury in the first place without a tourniquet. What would you do?

Ms. South: If I know that the patient is a possible replant candidate, I would notify our plastic surgeon in the hospital or the replantation team of the impending arrival. Upon arrival of the patient, I would assess for shock and monitor his vital signs. IV fluids would be given according to the patient's needs. If the pressure dressings are adequate, I would not tamper with them. If they are not, additional dressings would be applied without removing the first. One of the important things to note is that a clean injury or a sharp injury patient represents a better candidate than the patient with a grossly contaminated avulsed limb.

We would, of course, include in our regimen tetanus toxoid and give human antitoxin if indicated. An appropriate antibiotic would be started. We would type and crossmatch 3 to 6 units of blood according to the standard replantation protocol. The protocol also calls for x-rays of the chest, the extremity and the amputated part.

Moderator: Is there any discussion regarding the removal of the tourniquet? Does anyone object to that?

Response from floor: I do not know that I object to it, but I am just interested in knowing why Mr. Asbury said he would remove it. I would think that if a member of his crew had applied it, apparently there was enough bleeding for him to make that decision, and I wonder why he would release the tourniquet and cause perhaps some additional hypovolemia from massive hemorrhage.

Mr. Asbury: First of all, it is a relatively clean amputation, and in my experience, these are often associated with little bleeding. I think Dr. Aprahamian had said somebody on the construction crew had put the tourniquet on. It has been my experience that people who are not medically trained believe that tourniquets are great for any bleeding. That is the reason we removed it.

Moderator: I do not think there is much of an indication for the use of a tourniquet in this type of injury. If the tourniquet is on, before you remove it, you must obtain control of the hemorrhage, and this can be obtained with some type of pressure dressing. Once you have done it, there is control, and with control, there is no need for the tourniquet.

Ms. South, suppose that you do not have a replantation team, and I would suspect there is a fair number of hospitals in the United States that don't. What do you do? What happens if you do not have a replantation team in your hospital?

Ms. South: In my area, the medics know that the University Hospitals do have a replantation team. In any event, we do have some plastic surgeons who do work with amputated parts, so I would simply call one of them.

Moderator: We have been stressing the fact that the individual who has the ultimate responsibility for determining whether the amputated part is replantable is the head of the replantation team. We have been advocating that the amputated part and the patient be taken to a hospital that either has a replantation service or to a hospital where the patient can be stabilized and then transferred to a replantation institution.

This is the last case and represents a 20-year-old male who was run over by an automobile or truck. There is some ecchymosis of his abdomen, chest and left shoulder. Mr. Asbury, would you give us the details at the scene of the accident?

Mr. Asbury: I shall describe the scene of the accident a little bit further. This is a 20-year-old male who works as an attendant at a truck stop. He was walking out from between two parked cars and into the path of a semitrailer that hit and ran over him at a speed of about 15 to 20 mph. The area in which the patient was found represents a large parking lot. There is significant traffic and noise. It had been raining earlier in the day, and the evening was cool. The patient is lying on his back and is unconscious. Our initial impression is that the patient is profoundly shocky. Pre-hospital care consisted of placing a cervical collar on the patient and placing him on a spine board. Once moved into a more stable and controlled environment, further examination showed the signs of a significant injury to the chest and abdomen. Vital signs were compatible with shock. We contacted the emergency room, and while en route to the hospital, we described the patient to them. The hospital ordered oxygen by face mask and esophageal airway control as needed. We were instructed that if the esophageal airway was to be used a nasogastric tube should also be placed. The MAST suit was placed and inflated. IV of Ringer's lactate was started with a large bore needle. Biomedical telemetry was attached, and vital signs were continually monitored during our 20-minute trip to the hospital.

Moderator: Mr. Asbury, what was your assessment? What was your impression of the individual's problem? Why did you put on a cervical collar? Under what conditions would you put on a MAST suit and not inflate it?

Mr. Asbury: To answer the first question, he had crush injuries to his pelvis, abdomen and chest.

Moderator: What will these do to the patient?

Mr. Asbury: There will be considerable bleeding into the free spaces and from solid organs. We will have to look for liver lacerations and ruptures, splenic, pancreatic and kidney lacerations, compromised ventilation, with hemopneumothorax.

Moderator: Why did you use the cervical collar?

Mr. Asbury: This patient was found unconscious following trauma. We don't know if there is an associated cervical injury.

Moderator: When would you put the MAST suit on and not inflate it?

Mr. Asbury: We would use the trouser in a patient with significant or multiple trauma but who clinically is stable. Pants would be inflated upon a physician's decision or on deterioration of the patient.

Moderator: Let us return to the question of the cervical collar. What are your indications for its use?

Mr. Asbury: We were taught that when the patient is unconscious and is a victim of traumatic injury we are to assume that he has a cervical injury.

Moderator: We instruct our paramedics and EMTs to use the cervical collar when there is any obvious head injury or any suspected head injury, and we suspect a head injury in anybody who is unconscious or who has multiple organ system involvement.

Ms. South, now the patient is coming to your institution. What happens now?

Ms. South: The best thing is to be prepared for the emergency. I would have laboratory, x-ray and respiratory therapy on standby. When the patient arrives, I would leave him on the backboard, assure an adequate airway and IV, and would supplement them as indicated. I would be prepared and would have available a setup for peritoneal lavage if it is needed as well as nasogastric tube and chest tubes. A Foley catheter would be inserted, documenting color and amount and removing samples for blood. Tetanus boosters would be provided.

Moderator: What are your indications for doing peritoneal lavage? Better still, when would you *not* do peritoneal lavage?

Ms. South: You are asking me to infringe on the realm of the physician. Of course, I enjoy doing that. Is the abdomen distended or is there rigidity?

Moderator: Perhaps I should give the answers myself since I am a physician. There are two indications under which I would not do a peritoneal lavage. First, I would not do it on anybody on whom I am going to operate. My rationale is that if I am going to operate I do not need the lavage. I have already made up my mind that I am going to look and doing the lavage is superfluous. Second, I would not do it on anybody on whom I am not going to operate. The rationale is that I have already made the decision that there is nothing there which requires surgery so to do the lavage is unnecessary and would carry with it unnecessary morbidity. I would do the lavage on all of the cases in which I am not sure. I am not sure of someone who comes in with a head injury who is unconscious and is unable to give me an adequate history and physical. Many of the unconscious, traumatized patients also have multiple trauma and peritoneal lavage would be indicated. Anyone who enters with a cervical spinal injury or some type of cord injury in which there is difficulty in performing an adequate physical assessment requires a peritoneal lavage. The third indication would be in those individuals in whom I suspect intraabdominal problems who may be going to the operating room for some other condition, i.e., treatment of soft tissue injuries and fractures. In that situation, I would prefer to do a peritoneal lavage, too.

The other question that I would ask you, Ms. South, relates to the Foley catheter. Let us assume that in the process of inserting the catheter you noticed some blood in the urethra, and in trying to pass the catheter, you found it would not enter the bladder. What would you do now?

Ms. South: In this 20-year-old patient, there could be numerous reasons for this and social disease would have to be considered along with spasm.

Moderator: One of the concerns that we try to tell our nurses in the emergency department is that people who come in with abdominal and pelvic trauma may have GU tract pathology. They may have sustained either an anterior or posterior urethral injury. That individual who has several drops of blood coming from his penis may have sustained an anterior urethral injury. If you suspect this, a urethrogram should be performed. If the catheter cannot pass, it may be that the posterior urethra is torn, and this can often be confirmed by performing a rectal examination. In the case of a posterior urethral tear, the prostate will not be in its normal position.

I would like to mention just a few things regarding x-rays. The question can be asked: When do we order x-rays on a multiple trauma patient and in what order? The concern still has to be with ABCs. The patient should be stable prior to obtaining them, that is to say, airway management has been initiated and airway control is obtained. Respiratory assistance is being provided as indicated. IVs are in, and major fractures and cervical spinal injuries are stabilized. When the patient is stable, I believe the first x-ray that should be ordered and obtained is the cervical spine, following which an upright chest and KUB can be taken. If there are any suspicious findings, other ancillary x-rays employing contrast media can be performed. If the patient is noted to have significant respiratory difficulty, then a chest film is obtained first, followed by the cervical spine.

Panel: Initial Assessment and Resuscitation

Mary Beth Skelton, R.N.
Frank Lewis, Jr., M.D.
Don M. Benson, M.D.
Margaret M. Stevens, R.N., B.S.N.

Introduction

Mary Beth Skelton, R.N.

Initial assessment of the patient who presents to the emergency department usually falls on the emergency department nurse. The result of the nurse's initial assessment frequently exerts a significant influence on the quality of care that the patient subsequently receives. Physical manifestations of problems that might be overlooked in a busy emergency department can be recognized by a perceptive emergency department nurse. One must learn to obtain key information in a limited period of time and couple it with experienced observations. Initial steps of assessment of every patient coming into the emergency department should be based on a mental check list of observations that is followed consistently time after time.

The steps in initial assessment that are of prime importance are to (1) evaluate the level of consciousness; (2) evaluate the patency of the airway and the effectiveness of the ventilations and (3) evaluate the cardiovascular status of the patient.

Secondary assessment occurs when the initial life-threatening problems have been stabilized. Attention is then turned to identifying other injuries or signs and symptoms of illness. Secondary assessment also involves the repeated evaluation of the patient's vital signs as well as repeated evaluation of the initial injuries or signs and symptoms of illness.

Mary Beth Skelton, R.N., Director of Paramedic Training, Department of Surgery, Tulane University School of Medicine, New Orleans, La.; Member, Board of Directors, American Trauma Society.

Restoration of Blood Pressure

Frank Lewis, Jr., M.D.

Objectives

At the end of this paper the reader should have a knowledge of:

1. The appropriate immediate approach to developing intravenous access to severely injured patients.
2. The choices of intravenous solutions available and when to use them in critical situations.
3. The basic parameters to follow during volume resuscitation of patients critically injured.

I will discuss two elements regarding blood pressure because, in my experience caring for trauma victims at San Francisco General Hospital, I think these are most important in the initial treatment of hypovolemic patients: (1) route of access to the venous system and (2) fluid administration.

Route of Access

As in many other situations in the emergency department, this is a controversial subject. The problem is that upon initial examination of the patient, the picture presented may not be indicative of the true extent of injury. This can result from numerous causes. A patient with a very severe injury, if he reaches you quickly, may look fairly good initially and yet may have sustained massive visceral injury which will be lethal subsequently. So trying to determine blood loss from the initial examination of the patient is hazardous. If you see the patient three or four hours later and he is still doing well, is not shocky

---

Frank Lewis, Jr., M.D., Associate Professor of Surgery; Surgical Director, Intensive Care Unit, San Francisco General Hospital, Calif.; Founding Member, American Trauma Society.

and his perfusion is good, you can be fairly confident that he is not going to exsanguinate. But if you see him after ten minutes and he has a gunshot wound to the abdomen and he looks good, you cannot be at all certain of that. So with initial treatment, you have to put in lines for venous access that will allow the patient to be transfused massively, should it develop that he has major abdominal injury.

From the surgeon's viewpoint, the difficulty is that he no longer has access to the venous system once he has the patient in the operating room, opens the abdomen and begins to deal with whatever injuries he finds. When the drapes are on, you cannot get to the ankle or to the arm very well to put in a cutdown. You must put percutaneous lines in the neck, and they are not very big. So in the emergency department initial placement of venous access lines is critical in the later treatment of the patient. After you open the abdomen and decompress a massive source of blood loss, the anesthesiologist cannot rapidly transfuse the patient without large-bore IV lines, and you will lose the patient on the operating table.

The method of access available to you is basically either percutaneous or by cutdown. We feel that if a patient presents in any degree of shock, he should have a cutdown. We also feel strongly that the placement of percutaneous subclavian lines in the emergency department is a bad idea because it is associated with a significant incidence of pneumothorax. In the series where it has been examined, the incidence of pneumothorax is at least 10% to 15% from subclavian line placement. If you do that on all arrivals in the emergency department, you are going to worsen their condition. If, in a patient where it is already difficult to accurately assess the degree of injury, you give a pneumothorax as a result of your subclavian puncture, you only complicate the issue and compound the problem with which you are already trying to deal.

Internal jugular punctures in the emergency department are probably safer because, if done from the high approach, the chance of getting a pneumothorax is small. If done from the low approach, between the heads of the sternomastoid, it is about the same as subclavian and pneumothorax can result. Both problems can be avoided by doing cutdowns or by inserting peripheral lines.

If we see a patient who is not in shock and does not immediately show evidence of massive blood loss, we would be content with one large-bore peripheral line, something of the order of a large Intracath. However, if the patient presents in shock, then we feel a cutdown with tubing the size of standard IV tubing is mandatory because you do not know with what you are dealing. The largest region that you cannot assess immediately is the abdomen. You can assess what is occurring in the chest by the chest x-ray and by the placement of a chest tube to monitor blood loss, if the x-ray shows evidence of hemothorax. External bleeding from the extremities or the scalp is obviously monitored quite easily by looking at the patient. But you cannot see what is occurring in the abdomen until it is opened. You can sequester 2 liters of blood there without seeing any significant distention. Thus, you cannot rely upon physical examination of the injured patient to tell you how much bleeding there is within the abdomen. Treat the patient initially in a way that will handle all possibilities.

We prefer to do cutdowns at the ankle because the anatomy is so constant here. The greater saphenous vein passes just anterior to the medial malleolus and is so very consistent you can always find it there. Unless a patient has had a previous cutdown at that site, you can be assured of a vein into which you can insert a line. Slip a ligature around the vein distally, open it and insert a tube directly. The lines that we normally use are pediatric feeding tubes, 8 French size, or cutoff extension tubing. Typically we take regular IV extension tubing, cut off the distal end and slide it into the vein. That provides a big-bore line. If you need to pump blood rapidly, you can pump a unit of blood through a line that size in two or three minutes. You cannot do that through any percutaneous catheter. If you insert a large Intracath, the best you can do is pump blood in at a rate of about 1 unit every eight to ten minutes. That is hard to do. Therefore, if the patient is bleeding massively, percutaneous lines are inadequate. You need something the size of IV tubing.

Occasionally poor technique is a problem. This usually takes place in the rush and frenzy of resuscitation of patients who come in exsanguinated. In that situation, it is probably justified. But in most other situations, it is not. Take the time to do some sterile prep and put some towels around it to avoid the later complications of phlebitis. If you do cutdowns under these conditions, then they should be taken out within 12 to 24 hours. We prefer to do cutdowns in the antecubital fossa because you can thread the tubing centrally and get a central venous pressure out of it as well as a large-bore access line.

One procedure which I think is badly done in most emergency departments, and I do not really know why this particular belief ever got started, is that cutdowns in the arm must be done on the medial side of the arm and not directly in the antecubital fossa. This creates unnecessary difficulty. When you do it on the medial side of the arm, you must go down through the fascia of the arm, and it is very difficult to distinguish the brachial vein from the brachial artery in the patient who is exsanguinated. Where you cannot feel a pulse, you can easily mistake the brachial vein for the brachial artery. These problems can be avoided by going to the antecubital fossa, where the veins already stand out. You can get to them quite easily and can insert just as large a catheter there as with a medial cutdown. So in my opinion that is the preferred route.

Fluid Administration

It is fundamentally important to understand that if there is inadequate cardiac output, there are only two influencing factors: heart rate and stroke volume. You cannot do anything about heart rate. If the patient is young and has the ability to accelerate his heart rate, he will compensate whenever he is hypovolemic. Older patients cannot do this. As the patient gets older, heart rate is not as rapid in response to hypovolemia as in younger patients.

On the other hand, you do have some influence over stroke volume. The one thing you can most easily influence is the preload. You can provide volume for the patient to have adequate cardiac filling and, therefore, adequate ejection. You also can do something about contractility by administering inotropic agents, but that should be done only after the patient has had adequate preload, that is, he has had his vascular "tank" filled when he comes in and is hypovolemic.

What kind and how much fluid? The type of fluid has perhaps been overemphasized and the controversies that surround this area are unwarranted. By and large, in the emergency department, it probably does not make a great deal of difference what is used. There are many choices. With crystalloid solution, you can use isotonic saline or you can use any of the variety of balanced salt solutions. Among the crystalloid group, the only reason for choosing between isotonic sodium chloride and Ringer's lactate is because of the volume of infusion that you may give the patient. Otherwise, there is really no difference between these two solutions. There was a very good evaluation study conducted during the Vietnam War. The only difference demonstrated was that the patients who received saline had higher chlorides a day or so later. Otherwise, there was no difference in resuscitative effects. Do not lose sight of the fact that either solution will work in the hypovolemic patient. The main difference occurs upon infusion of massive volumes of crystalloid solution (5 or 6 liters in 30 minutes) to an exsanguinated patient. In that situation, if you replace with saline, then you are giving the patient much more chloride than he normally has present and somewhat more sodium. Therefore, over a period of very rapid resuscitation, he will become hyperchloremic and will have to compensate for that later by renal excretion. That is not a tremendous problem, but it does give him more of an acid load to excrete. The sodium concentration in saline is 154 mEq as opposed to 140 mEq in the normal serum, so it is a little high. The chloride concentration in saline is 154 mEq as opposed to 100 mEq to 105 mEq in the normal serum, about 50% higher than normal serum. The only advantage of the balanced salt solutions is that they more closely approximate normal human plasma. Ringer's lactate has 129 mEq of sodium, 28 mEq of bicarbonate and 101 mEq of chloride. Therefore, when giving massive volumes of crystalloid over a short period, if you give Ringer's lactate, you are not going to change the electrolyte concentration in his serum very much. You are certainly going to dilute out the red cell concentration and make him anemic, but you will not change the ionic composition. Therefore, you will not generate secondary problems related to these ionic changes. Any of these products are equivalent, in my opinion, that are listed under balanced salt solutions: Ringer's lactate, Ringer's acetate, Plasmanate, Normosol, or any of the other variety of solutions that are made commercially today.

The only situation which I think does deserve some consideration is when you are going to transfuse the crystalloid solution and you are subsequently going to put blood up in the same line. If you use solutions that contain calcium, and the Ringer solutions are the only ones that do, you can get hemolysis and/or coagulation of blood from the addition of calcium to the blood before it gets into the patient. That is fairly uncommon, but it has been shown to be an unequivocal problem in some situations.

The objection to Ringer's lactate is that, in fact, you are giving lactic acid or lactate, which gives the patient an effect like lactic acid. To me this is not a problem. Many people have studied this and have never been able to demonstrate that it has any effect whatsoever in patients who have been resuscitated from hypovolemic shock. Lactate is converted to bicarbonate in a single pass through the liver. Basically, the crystalloid solutions are equivalent, except when massive administration is necessary, and then one of the balanced salt solutions is probably better than normal saline.

In terms of the colloids which are available, various types of blood can be obtained, depending upon the blood bank in your own hospital. Our preference is for type-specific blood rather than low-titer or O-negative. There are fewer adverse reactions to this. The best situation, of course, is to have fully typed and cross-matched blood. But if blood is required rapidly for transfusion, that may not be possible. It takes about an hour to get a full cross-match. If you want type-specific blood, your chance of having a reaction will be less than 5%, and it will be slightly higher with low-titer or negative. That will vary somewhat in your own specific locale, as to what is available. In the future, washed red cells or frozen red cells that have been reconstituted may become more available. Currently in our area, that technology has not been developed to the point of practicality.

Perhaps available in the future are the stroma-free hemoglobin solutions for direct transfusion of hemoglobin, rather than red cells. There is some very promising work going on in that area, but it is not yet clinically available.

Under the other colloid solutions, plasma and the various ways in which it is given all are roughly equivalent, either fresh frozen plasma, concentrated albumin or Plasmanate solutions, or any of the other commercially available ones which are equivalent. Basically, all you are giving with those is 4% protein plus a balanced salt solution. The principal effect of the plasma solutions is giving volume to the patient in the form of a salt solution. The protein that goes along with it has relatively few effects. Certain situations in which it really makes a difference, those effects are probably harmful. Plasma substitutes, such as Dextran, can be used but they are limited in volume. If you give more than 1,000 cc of either clinical or low molecular weight Dextran, bleeding problems from paralysis of the platelet system may occur. So these are really of little use in the resuscitation of the trauma patient where you already have a bleeding problem if you need volume replacement. We do not advocate the use of Dextran at all.

The real question in use of protein vs. crystalloid solutions concerns one of expense. About one year ago 250 cc of Plasmanate cost about $40. The cost may have risen slightly by now. If you use concentrated albumin, it is about the same for 50 cc. On the other hand, Ringer's lactate costs about 1/20th as much for a 1-liter solution. Therefore, if you get the same effect from crystalloid and it costs much less and the Plasmanate does nothing specifically beneficial, why use it? Therefore, we do not use it. For the past ten years, in emergency patients at San Francisco General Hospital, we have never used Plasmanate and we very rarely use it even within the hospital. We feel that crystalloid replacement is equivalent in most of these patients. In the rare instances when we really need to give protein, we can obtain and administer it. But it is probably more effective, even in those situations, to give the patient amino acids in the form of hyperalimentation and let the patient make his own protein.

Indices of Successful Resuscitation

One critical indicator is the return of the urine output to at least 0.5 cc/kg/hr, so that a 70-kg man would excrete about 35 cc. That is a minimal amount. We really feel more comfortable if we see twice that much. Another critical indicator is adequate peripheral perfusion. I think this is one of the least emphasized things that is available to you just standing at the side of the patient. We place relatively little emphasis on blood pressure per se. Of all the indicators in following a patient who is being resuscitated, blood pressure would be about fifth on the list I would be interested in seeing. The first is skin perfusion and this is something you can assess quickly and easily just by putting your hand on the patient. If the patient's skin is moist and pale and he is constricted, then you have not given him enough volume. Once the patient is adequately resuscitated, the moistness disappears because the epinephrine that he is elaborating to compensate disappears. His skin becomes pinker, warmer and drier. Simply feeling the skin is one of the easiest and best methods to tell whether you have been successful. Peripheral perfusion and urine output together are the two most critical factors to observe. If a central venous line is in, it is comforting to know that the patient's atrial filling pressures have been restored to near normal. It is nice to have that measurement because of the possibility of tension pneumothorax or pericardial tamponade, but it is not critical in the resuscitation of every patient.

Return of the patient's mental status, assuming no head injury, to an alert and oriented situation is indicative of successful resuscitation and perfusion of the head. It is possible that in the future direct monitoring of cardiac output will be of some value, but we do not do it now because we do not place Swan-Ganz catheters in the emergency department. Rather, we wait and do that in the intensive care unit. In the emergency situation, we feel that CVP is adequate for following these patients.

When you observe the results of your resuscitation, if there is adequate urine output and if the CVP or wedge pressure seems to be high, then you should decrease the fluid administration. That is simply telling you that you are overdoing it and should cut back a bit and let the patient diurese. If the urine output and CVP or wedge pressure are low, then you need to speed up your fluid administration and try to catch up with the patient and find out why he is losing it and why you are not ahead of him. The real problem comes here, when you have a high filling pressure and a low urine output, because the question then becomes: What has gone wrong? What are the problems that you need to deal with? In this situation, knowing cardiac output is of tremendous benefit because, on the one hand, the principal problem that you have to deal with is cardiac and, on the other hand, renal. If there is low cardiac output in that situation, then you need to assess myocardial function directly and see what the problem is that is causing the low cardiac output. On the other hand, if cardiac output is high in that situation, there is probably a problem with the kidney and you need to assess renal function in the form of the concentrating mechanism, serum/urine creatinine ratios, creatinine clearance and free water clearance, to determine whether the patient already is developing acute renal failure.

If the problem is cardiac output, you need to deal with whatever is causing it, possibly using inotropic agents. If the problem is in the kidney, and the patient is developing ATN, then the use of an osmotic diuretic may have some effect in ameliorating the renal failure which results.

In normal hemorrhagic shock of moderate to mild degree, there is no evidence that any sort of a capillary leak or a change in capillary permeability is produced in the body. On the other hand, there is some experimental evidence in animals that shows that in severe hemorrhagic shock or prolonged hemorrhagic shock, a capillary leak may occur and the pore size or the effective pore size in the capillary may enlarge, so that the capillaries begin to leak protein solutions which they normally would not do. In this situation, then, the type of fluid administered should be based upon physiologic principles as to what is occurring. The situation you have is that, in the capillary, if you have a leak, the normal colloid pressure in the interstitium will be raised significantly by the administration of protein-containing solutions. In that situation, crystalloid solutions are far more beneficial than any of the protein-containing solutions, such as albumin or Plasmanate. Therefore, in the situation where you have very severe or very prolonged shock, Plasmanate-containing solutions are probably harmful, and crystalloid solutions are far better. In the average patient with mild to moderate shock, it probably does not make any difference and the decision should be made on the basis of expense.

Self-Evaluation Quiz

1. The most important step one must take to increase perfusion when treating a patient with severe trauma and hypotension is:
   a) Insert large-bore peripheral venous lines
   b) Type and cross 6 units of blood
   c) EKG and CXR
   d) Examination of fundi
   e) Subclavian line placement
2. The ideal location for cutdowns for large-bore IV catheters is:
   a) Subclavian
   b) Ankle or antecubital fossa
   c) Medial side of arm
   d) Brachiocephalic vein
   e) Femoral vein
3. In maintaining adequate perfusion of tissue there must be:
   a) Adequate cardiac output
   b) Adequate intravascular volume
   c) Sufficient cardiac filling
   d) The urine output and skin temperature are good monitoring indices
   e) All of the above
4. One of the benefits of Ringer's lactate over normal saline in massive infusion:
   a) It provides lactate
   b) It is a hypotonic solution
   c) Massive volumes over short periods do not alter electrolyte balance
   d) It is high in carbohydrates
   e) All of the above
5. Many recommend using normal saline rather than Ringer's in patients who may require transfusion because:
   a) It requires less tubing
   b) The calcium in Ringer's may coagulate or hemolyze blood
   c) Ringer's is hypotonic
   d) There is less chance for infection
   e) None of the above

6. Ringer's lactate more closely resembles human plasma for its:
   a) Sodium concentration is 129 mEq
   b) Chloride concentration is 154 mEq
   c) Chloride concentration is 101 mEq
   d) Na concentration is 154 mEq
   e) a and c
   f) b and d
7. Colloid solutions are basically 4% protein and a balanced salt solution.
   a) True
   b) False

Answers on page 289.

Emergency Oxygenation, Ventilation and Airway Control in the Trauma Victim

Don M. Benson, M.D.

Objectives

1. To state the three goals of airway control, which of the three should receive priority and reasons for same.
2. To describe the two general categories of airway control techniques, including the advantages and disadvantages of each.
3. To discuss the diagnosis of partial and complete upper airway obstruction in breathing and nonbreathing patients.
4. To distinguish between upper and lower airway obstruction.
5. To list in order of application the steps to be followed in approaching the victim of airway compromise.
6. To describe the contraindications, if any, of each step.
7. To discuss the role of tracheostomy in emergency airway control.

Introduction

There are three goals of airway control: (1) oxygenation, (2) ventilation and (3) protection of the lungs from soilage.

A maximally effective approach to the trauma victim with airway compromise requires review of basic anatomic and physiologic principles.

The function of the airway is to provide a path for delivery of oxygen-containing gas to the lungs' respiratory exchange surfaces. There oxygen is loaded onto transport units (hemo-

Don M. Benson, M.D., Clinical Associate Professor of Anesthesiology, University of Pittsburgh; Medical Director, Stark County Paramedic Training Program, Canton, Ohio.

globin molecules). From there oxygen is moved to the tissues and cells where it participates in generation of high energy compounds essential for life processes.

During periods of low or absent oxygen delivery, generation of high energy compounds is retarded, but it does not stop instantaneously. Vital processes continue precariously for a short time before grinding to a halt and terminating permanently hope for revival.

The principal, maximally urgent, overriding responsibility of the resuscitist when faced with airway compromise is re-oxygenation. The resuscitist must before all else strive to meet metabolic oxygen demands to whatever extent possible.

The amount of oxygen delivered to body tissues is described by the term oxygen transport. Oxygen transport is the product of cardiac output (L/min) and oxygen content (vol%). Oxygen content is the product of 1.34* × Hbg concentration × % saturation of hemoglobin by oxygen plus 0.003† × paO_2.

Oxygen transport can be increased by increasing cardiac output, all other things being equal. The sigmoid shape of the oxyhemoglobin saturation curve permits increases of the oxygen content by increasing the paO_2. Small increases in paO_2 can result in substantial increase in the percent saturation of hemoglobin in hypoxic states. For instance, a paO_2 of 23 torr results in a hemoglobin saturation of 40%. Raising the paO_2 only 3 torr, to 26 torr, results in an increase in SaO_2 to 50%.

Raising the paO_2 from 23 torr to 45 torr doubles the oxyhemoglobin saturation raising it from 40% to 80%.

The importance of this observation lies in the fact that in the emergency situation increasing the inspired oxygen concentration often raises the paO_2 and this in turn raises the SaO_2.

Even in the face of a very significant partial airway obstruction, the resuscitist can gain precious seconds and forestall the calamitous consequences of tissue hypoxia by increasing the inspired oxygen concentration. While equipment is being assembled, while a plan is being formed to cope with the underlying problem, while higher level consultants are being

*1.34 ml of O_2 per gram of fully saturated hemoglobin.

†0.003 ml of O_2 dissolved per ml plasma per torr partial pressure oxygen.

mobilized, the critical component of the asphyxial process — hypoxia — can be treated by increasing the inspired oxygen concentration. Even a small increase can result in a sizable increase in the saturation of hemoglobin by oxygen and thus in turn result in a sizable increase in oxygen transport. The first priority in airway control must always be re-oxygenation.

The second goal of airway control is pulmonary ventilation. As oxygen is consumed in the metabolic processes generating high energy bonds, carbon dioxide is generated. Carbon dioxide is transported to the pulmonary gas exchange surface and by the mechanical processes of lung ventilation is moved to the outside. Failure of pulmonary ventilation with accumulation of carbon dioxide will lead to respiratory acidosis and, eventually, after many hours or days to death. This process, unlike hypoxia, is not fatal in seconds to minutes. It must be corrected, but not with the urgency that hypoxia must be corrected.

The third component of airway control is protection of the tracheobronchial tree from soilage by foreign matter.

Contamination of the tracheobronchial tree can result in a number of problems, namely, obstruction of conducting airways, bronchospasm alteration of ratio of alveolar ventilation to dead space ventilation, increase of physiologic shunt, pulmonary inflammation and/or infection. All can occur with varying degrees of severity. The consequences of pulmonary aspiration can cause death, but not with the potential rapidity of hypoxia. The resuscitist faced with the agonizing choice of attempting to prevent tracheobronchial soilage in the face of rapidly progressive hypoxia or permitting pulmonary aspiration while re-oxygenating must give priority to re-oxygenation.

Lest I be misunderstood, let me elaborate and give examples.

Case 1

A previously healthy 22-year-old man comes to the emergency room having sustained blunt injury of the anterior chest wall as a result of being thrown against a steering wheel in an automobile accident. The patient is stuporous but responsive. Cervical spine fracture has been ruled out, but the patient has a very significant flail chest wall. You expose the larynx transorally and just as you place the tip of the endotracheal tube at the laryngeal introitus, gastric contents well up from the esophagus into the hypopharynx.

Case 2

You are called to the emergency department to assist in the care of a 53-year-old man who has sustained an open fracture of the left femur, tibia and fibula as a result of a motorcycle accident. The patient is alert but complaining of severe retrosternal crushing pain radiating to his left arm. He is pale and diaphoretic. As you assess the situation, he lapses into unconsciousness, has a grand mal seizure and then becomes limp, pulseless and apneic. CPR is begun. The patient regurgitates large volumes of liquid and semisolid gastric contents.

Analysis of Airway Control Problems in Above Cases

The most rapid method of improving oxygenation in the first case is rapid completion of the tracheal intubation, isolation of the trachea from the vomitus by inflating the endotracheal tube cuff and ventilation via the endotracheal tube with an oxygen-rich gas mixture.

In the second case, however, a few seconds or perhaps minutes will be required before the equipment required for transoral tracheal intubation can be made ready. Therefore, the resuscitist should at least partially clear the airway with whatever means available and ventilate the patient with an oxygen-rich mixture while assistants prepare intubation equipment. Only after all necessary equipment is immediately ready should ventilation/oxygenation be interrupted to intubate the trachea.

These two cases are relatively clear cut. In both cases, priority goes to oxygenation. Clinical situations are seldom so obvious. Judgment is required. The key matter to remember is the top priority of oxygenation. Ventilation and protection from airway soilage are urgent and should be accomplished as quickly as reasonably possible, but not at the unnecessary expense of oxygenation.

Diagnosis of Airway Obstruction

Many times airway compromise is obvious. A patient shot in the face, gasping, coughing large amounts of blood, along with bone fragments, teeth and other unidentifiable tissue obviously is a victim of airway compromise. Other times it is more subtle. A patient comatose from close head injury lies quietly, silently aspirating regurgitated gastric contents.

When confronted with a patient possibly having airway obstruction, the first determination one must make is the presence or absence of breathing movement. Examine the chest and abdominal walls for movement. If breathing movements are present, assess their adequacy. If you are in doubt as to the adequacy of the spontaneous tidal volume or obviously if it is absent, begin the airway control sequences described below.

If the patient's spontaneous tidal volume appears to be adequate, determine the presence or absence of inspirating soft tissue retractions (i.e., retractions of the suprasternal notch, supraclavicular areas or intercostal space). Presence of such retractions indicates a disparity between inspiratory intrapulmonary and ambient pressure. Such disparity can be caused either by partial or complete upper airway obstruction and/or inadequate intercostal muscle function. If the patient is experiencing partial upper airway obstruction, snoring or gurgling may be heard. Regardless of the cause, actions described below are indicated.

When confronted with an apneic patient, immediately launch into the airway control steps described below. If airway obstruction is not a significant component of the patient's problem, attempts to ventilate will be successful. If the airway is obstructed, attempts to ventilate will be met with obvious resistance. Again, the course of action is described below.

When examining a spontaneously breathing conscious patient with chest wall soft tissue retraction, one must differentiate between partial upper airway obstruction and partial lower airway obstruction — for example, asthma. The history may be helpful. Patients with upper airway obstruction will have a history of acute recent onset, while patients with partial lower airway obstruction will probably have a history of prior occurrences, possibly aggravated by allergies or respiratory tract infections. The management of lower airway obstruction includes bronchodilators, infection control and other treatment beyond the scope of our present discussion.

Airway Control Techniques

Airway control techniques are divided into two categories — those requiring cannulation of the trachea and those not requiring cannulation of the airway. Noncannulating techniques are easy to learn, noninvasive and effective but have certain drawbacks, viz. lack of protection against tracheal soilage and failure to create a gas-tight fit between the ventilation device and the conducting airway. Lack of a gas-tight fit between ventilation device and trachea limits effective inspiratory pressure to esophageal opening pressure. Cannulating techniques are more difficult to learn and require physical invasion of the patient's airway but do provide aspiration protection and permit a gas-tight connection between the ventilation device and the conducting airway so high inspiratory pressures can be used if needed.

Noncannulating Airway Control Steps

1. *Head tilt.* In unconsciousness all of the muscles of the body become limp. The tongue, being a muscle, also becomes limp. In the supine patient the tongue is pulled by gravity into the posterior hypopharynx and obstructs the breathing passage. Since the tongue is attached to the anterior cervical tissues, it can often be displaced away from the posterior pharyngeal wall by simply stretching the anterior neck tissues. This is easily accomplished by tilting the head on the occipito-atlantal junction. Head tilt is effectively accomplished by placing one hand under the neck and the other hand on the forehead. The hand under the neck lifts upward and the hand on the forehead pushes downward, thus moving the head into position of extension. The anterior cervical tissues are stretched, the tongue is pulled away from the back of the throat and the airway is cleared. This maneuver alone will alleviate airway obstruction in approximately 80% of the cases.

This maneuver is contraindicated in suspected neck injury and relatively contraindicated in infants where excessive hyperextension will cause collapse of the soft cartilaginous tracheal rings. Excessive or aggressive snapping of the neck backward during this maneuver may cause physical injury to the cervical spine; therefore, it should be carried out quite gently.

2. *Chin lift.* Guildner (*JACEP* 5 (8):598, 1976) described the chin lift maneuver. The fingers of one hand are placed under the lower jaw on the chin. The chin is lifted forward, supporting the jaw and helping tilt the head backward. With the other hand the forehead is pressed downward tilting the head backward. The thumb of the hand under the chin may be used to lightly depress the lower lip. The teeth should be nearly brought together by the hand lifting the chin. Guildner found the chin lift was more effective and more easily learned than the neck lift or jaw thrust (see below) in controlling upper airway obstruction. If intermittent positive pressure ventilation (IPPV) is required while using the chin lift maneuver, it can be applied in the conventional way, using the thumb and index finger of the hand on the forehead to pinch the nose.

3. *IPPV (with oxygen, if possible).* Some oxygenation can be accomplished even in the partially obstructed airway by increasing the pressure gradient across the obstruction. The mouth must be open for exhalation, since 20% of the patients cannot exhale through the nose. (The soft palate swings cephalad, obstructing the internal nares thus prohibiting exhalation through the nose.) IPPV may be performed using the mouth to mouth or mouth to nose technique or with a positive pressure ventilation device (self-refilling bag, valve mask unit) if available.

If laryngospasm (spasm of the extrinsic laryngeal muscles) is present when IPPV is attempted, the laryngospasm will be worsened instead of inproved unless the next maneuver (forward displacement of the mandible) is also applied.

4. *Forward displacement of the mandible*

a. *Primary technique (triple airway maneuver).* Take a position behind the victim's head looking over his nose toward his toes and curve both index fingers as though pulling triggers on guns. Place the radial aspect of your index fingers on the ascending rami of the mandible, identified easily by palpitating the mandible in the vicinity of the ear lobes. Place your thumbs at the junction of the anterior and middle thirds of the mandible. Three maneuvers are then carried out. First, the mandible is rotated downward to open the mouth. Second, the mandible is displaced forward by raising it toward the ceiling, i.e., the radial aspects of index fingers are used to raise the mandible while the rotational movement of the wrist moves the anterior portion of the mandible toward the toes. Third, the head is extended on the occipito-atlantal junction as the mandible is lifted toward the ceiling. In sum, the three maneuvers are (1) forward displacement of the mandible, (2) opening the mouth and (3) tilting the head backward. These maneuvers will open the airway in well over 95% of obstructed patients.

b. *Alternate technique — for use in deeply comatose patients.* In deeply comatose patients the risk of being bitten is nonexistent. The same anatomic effect can be accomplished as described above, by simply grasping the mandible between the thumb and index finger and pulling it firmly toward the ceiling.

In either maneuver IPPV can be applied using the mouth to mouth or mouth to nose method. Remember to seal the patient's nose when using mouth to mouth breathing. If both hands are in use, seal the nose with your cheek.

The vicious cycle of laryngospasm can be broken with the triple airway maneuver. As the mandible is lifted upward, the epiglottis is displaced upward, thus allowing gas or the rescuer's exhaled air under positive pressure to be forced under it and into the larynx and trachea.

5. *Foreign body removal.* Foreign bodies can be solid or nonsolid. Since the resuscitative approach differs, we shall examine each independently:

a. *Nonsolid (liquid or semiliquid) foreign bodies.* Regurgitation of gastric contents may flood the hypopharynx and trachea with liquid, semisolid material frequently containing particles of small to moderate sizes, i.e., not large enough to obstruct the larynx.

The liquid material can be removed from the mouth by suctioning, if available. The suction source should be capable of generating high flow rates and vacuum. Tubing should be nonkinkable and a rigid tonsil suction tip should be used, since it is far more easily directed than is a nonrigid catheter.

In the absence of suction apparatus, the mouth can be swept with the rescuer's finger or blotted with the patient's bed clothes.

If the patient is on a long, 6-foot spine immobilization board, it can be moved into a steep head down position by raising the foot end approximately 3 feet off the ground. This maneuver places the larynx higher than the posterior hypopharynx and may help protect the trachea from soilage.

Observing hundreds of milliliters of gastric contents welling up in the mouth of an unconscious patient is an alarming experience. Rapid suction is required to help prevent a catastrophe. However, while the action must be prompt, it cannot be without thought. For instance, if the patient has an unstable cervical spine fracture, rapid rotation of the head and suctioning of the mouth may prevent or reduce aspiration only at the expense of inducing quadraplegia. Well-intentioned but thoughtless reflex attempts to roll a vomiting patient onto his side may be counterproductive if a previously placed but unnoticed endotracheal tube is dislocated. As with all aspects of airway control, regurgitation and threatened tracheal soilage must be managed with aggression, effectiveness but, most important, forethought.

b. *Solid matter.* The *conscious patient* typically is very young (under 4 years of age) or relatively old (over 50 years). In the older age group, the patient typically is edentulous or has poorly fitting dentures, has been consuming alcoholic beverages and is in a festive setting. The patient inhales a piece of food. He experiences distress and grabs his neck with his hand. This has become known as a universal distress sign. The rescuer should ask the patient, who will usually at that point be standing, "Can you talk?" If the victim shakes his head no, foreign body food impaction in the larynx must be suspected and treatment applied. The rescuer positions himself behind the patient. He places both arms around the patient so that his hands come to rest in the epigastrium midway between xiphoid and the umbilicus. The rescuer makes a fist with one hand and grasps that fist with the other hand. The clenched fist is then given an abrupt jerk in a direction toward the upper thoracic spine, thus causing an abrupt rise in intrathoracic pressure. This "artificial cough maneuver" is repeated four times. If this fails to displace the impacted food, the rescuer gives four sharp blows between the shoulder blades and again repeats the artificial cough maneuver. This sequence is repeated until the foreign body is extracted or until the patient lapses into unconsciousness. If the patient becomes unconscious he is placed supine on the floor and the protocol given below is continued.

In the *unconscious patient* suspected of having foreign body food impaction I recommend the following procedure.

1. Tilt the head.
2. Provide IPPV.
3. If unsuccessful, apply forward displacement of mandible and again attempt positive pressure ventilation.
4. If unsuccessful, open the mouth using the crossed finger maneuver and sweep the mouth with the fingers of the other hand. The crossed finger maneuver is carried out by placing the index finger on the upper teeth and thumb on the lower teeth if the rescuer is above the patient's head. If the rescuer is at the side, the index finger is placed on the lower teeth and thumb on the upper teeth. In either event by crossing the thumb and index finger one can open the mouth by using the flexor muscles of the forearm. The flexor muscles are stronger than the extensors and have better mechanical advantage than do the extensors.

   The mouth is opened. The rescuer reaches inside with his fingers and with two or three brief, deep sweeping movements tries to extricate the foreign body. Most foreign body food impactions occur with a piece of meat or other material as large as a pack of cigarettes. It can frequently be reached from above by the thumb and index finger and extricated manually.
5. If unsuccessful, the victim is rolled toward the rescuer and four sharp blows are given between the shoulder blades. The patient is returned to a supine position where four chest compressions are given. The chest compressions are the same as those used in external compression. Airway pressures similar to those generated by the abdominal thrust maneuver are achieved with external cardiac compression without as much apparent risk of abdominal organ injury as with the abdominal thrust maneuver. Following that, the mouth is again swept and again head tilt and IPPV are attempted. If still unsuccessful the sequence is repeated until airway patency is established.

During this exercise it is important to realize that 100% airway obstruction is exceedingly rare. The victim may be 90% obstructed and by giving IPPV the pressure gradient across the obstruction is increased and some minor but crucial emergency re-oxygenation can be obtained.

One final word on foreign body removal. The method of choice is removal under direct vision. If an experienced rescuer (physician or paramedic) is available and has endoscopy equipment, the airway should be visualized and the obstructing mass removed with a foreign body forcep. If all other methods fail, these patients may be candidates for cricothyrotomy or transtracheal jet ventilation (see below).

6. *Oropharyngeal/nasopharyngeal airway.* An oropharyngeal or nasopharyngeal airway provides certain advantages. The hands of the rescuer are free to engage in additional airway control maneuvers and positive pressure ventilation. Properly inserted airways hold the tongue away from the posterior pharyngeal wall and help keep the mouth open, facilitating exhalation. They do not help prevent aspiration of foreign matter. In fact, they may aggravate the situation if used in too lightly an unconscious patient by stimulating gagging, retching and vomiting. In addition, an airway that is too short may impact against the base of the tongue, driving it into the larynx, thus compounding the airway obstruction rather than relieving it. Likewise, an airway that is too large can actually impact the epiglottis into the larynx, again compounding the airway obstruction rather than relieving it. Typically a medium or large adult airway will be satisfactory in most adult male patients.

The technique of oropharnygeal airway insertion is as follows: Standing at the patient's occiput, looking over his nose toward his toes, the rescuer opens the mouth using the crossed finger maneuver with the nondominant hand. With the dominant hand, the rescuer raises the base of the patient's tongue with a tongue blade. While the base of the tongue is being held up away from the posterior oropharynx, the dominant hand is used to pass an oropharyngeal airway into place. Care must be used to insure the airway is of proper size and the tongue and lips are not caught between the airway and the teeth.

Alternatively, the airway itself can be used to move the tongue away from the posterior oropharynx as follows. With the mouth being held open with the crossed finger maneuver, the airway is inserted into the mouth upside down, so the distal (nonflanged) end of the airway sweeps the base of the tongue away from posterior oropharyngeal airway. The airway is then rotated 180° to its final normal position. Again, be sure soft tissues are not trapped between the teeth and the airway.

Airway insertion is relatively simple, but as with most of the techniques described here, skill should be developed by practicing on a resuscitation mannikin or on an anesthetized human under careful supervision by an experienced operator.

The nasopharyngeal airway has many of the same advantages and disadvantages as the oropharyngeal airway. However, the nasopharyngeal is better tolerated in the lightly unconscious patient. The important things to remember in using a nasopharyngeal airway are to use a soft rubber nasal airway and to coat it generously with lubricating jelly.

Cannulating Airway Control Steps

1. *Esophageal obturator airway (EOA)/Esophagogastric tube airway (EGTA).* The EOA can be visualized as a large endotracheal tube with a plug in the end, a 35 cc cuff and holes drilled in the wall of the tube midway between the proximal and distal ends. The distal end of the EOA is fitted with a mask. The device is inserted into the esophagus by lifting the jaw and blindly pushing the instrument into the mouth. As the instrument is pushed deeply into the throat, a distal end enters the esophagus and comes to lie below the carina. The mask becomes seated firmly on the patient's face. The 35 cc balloon is inflated. The rescuer then provides positive pressure ventilation through the tube using whatever means available. Air is forced down the tube and out the holes midway between the proximal and distal ends of the tube. These holes will usually have come to lie in the vicinity of the laryngeal introitus. The patient is protected from regurgitation of gastric contents. However, the hypopharynx may still be obstructed by the patient's tongue; therefore, the use of the EOA must be accompanied by head tilt. In addition, potential problems include inadvertent tracheal insertion, difficulty in securing a gas-tight fit with the mask and tracheal soilage with foreign matter accumulated above the balloon (e.g., teeth, blood).

The EGTA is superior to the EOA in that the tube leading from the ambient atmosphere to the esophagus has been refitted with an open plug at the distal end so that the nasogastric tube can be passed through the tube into the stomach for decompression. In the EOA no such mechanism is available. Therefore, when the cuff is deflated and the EOA is removed, regurgitation of the gastric contents commonly occurs. If the trachea has not been protected from soilage, aspiration may occur.

In addition, the EGTA has been fitted with a different type of mask. The tube coming from the esophagus to the ambient atmosphere passes through a hole in the mask. A second hole in the mask is provided for positive pressure ventilation. The 35 cc balloon on the esophageal end of the tube creates a gas-tight system between the rescuer's positive pressure point and the remainder of the upper airway. Again, tracheal soilage with material from above is not prevented and the problems of soft tissue airway obstruction and mask leak to some extent remain.

When either the EOA or the EGTA is used, the trachea should be intubated prior to removal of the instrument, assuming, of course, the patient is still a victim of airway compromise.

2. *Orotracheal intubation/nasotracheal intubation.* The endotracheal tube provides ideal airway control. A gas-tight, aspiration resistant airway is secured.

While preparations are being made to intubate the trachea the patient should be oxygenated using non-cannulating airway techniques described above. The tracheal tube is passed in a conventional manner. Training in endotracheal intubation should be obtained under supervision of an anesthesiologist or a nurse anesthetist using anesthetized healthy patients.

In some circumstances nasotracheal intubation is preferred. Such circumstances prevail when neck movement is contraindicated (e.g., suspected cervical spine fracture).

Recently a new device has been introduced, the *Berman Airway.* The Berman Airway is an oropharyngeal airway with a very large internal lumen. In addition a slit is made in one side of the airway. There is also a short plastic extrusion on the distal end. Berman maintains the airway can be inserted in the usual manner as is an oropharyngeal airway. A tracheal tube can then be passed through the airway into the tracheal lumen blindly without additional instrumentation. The Berman Airway can then be removed if necessary by simply sliding the endotracheal tube out through the slit in the side of the airway. The author continues that if inadvertently esophageal intubation is accomplished, the rescuer need simply inflate the endotracheal tube balloon and he will have isolated the esophagus thus preventing the gastric aspiration. My personal experience with the Berman Airway has been less than fully satisfactory. The reader is encouraged to watch the literature for further evaluation of this device.

3. *Cricothyrotomy.* Cricothyrotomy must be considered an emergency re-oxygenation procedure to be performed by only surgically orientated physicians. The technique for right-handed operators is as follows:

The trachea is grasped between the thumb and the long finger of the left hand. The index finger of the left hand is used to palpate the thyroid cartilage, the cricoid ring and the intervening cricothyroid membrane. A scalpel or other knife blade is used to make a small incision in the skin over the cricothyroid membrane. Incision of skin is essential prior to inserting the cricothyroid membrane cannula for the following reason: the skin is the toughest tissue between the ambient atmosphere and the cervical spine. If one pushes a cannula with sufficient force to pass the skin, that force will also be great enough to drive the cannula through the subcutaneous tissue, the cricothyroid membrane, the posterior tracheal wall and the esophagus. The instrument will come to rest in the anterior cervical spine, creating in the process a tracheoesophageal fistula.

Having incised the skin, using a cricothyrotome (e.g., a beveled right angle tracheal tube adapter), one can blunt dissect through the subcutaneous tissues of the cricothyroid membrane into the tracheal lumen. Care must be taken to be sure the cannula does not lie in the pretracheal fascia. Positive pressure ventilation must then be given through the cannula whether or not the patient is breathing spontaneously since the tiny lumen of the cricothyroid cannula is far too small to permit sufficient ventilation to maintain life viability. Cricothyrotomy is an alternative only until surgical tracheostomy or orotracheal intubation can be performed.

Complications include pretracheal fascia bleeding, inadvertent laceration of the thyroid, pneumothorax and pneumomediastinum. I do not recommend cricothyrotomy for general use. It is included here only for completeness. Efforts should be concentrated on perfecting noncannulating upper airway control techniques. An alternative to cricothyrotomy is given below.

4. *Transtracheal jet ventilation.* The cricothyroid membrane is traversed with a catheter over a needle-type cannula (e.g., Angiocath). Again, the skin must be incised with a scalpel prior to inserting the catheter. Having entered the tracheal lumen (established by free aspiration of air from the cannula with a syringe), the steel needle is removed and the plastic cannula is left in situ. An anesthesia extension tube is connected to the cannula proximally and distally to a three way plastic stopcock. The second part of the stopcock is connected to an oxygen delivery tube which goes directly to a 50 PSI oxygen source. A flowmeter is not placed between the oxygen source and the cannula. One then directs one-second bursts of oxygen into the cannula interspersing it with two-second periods for exhalation to the cannula.

This technique does not allow for exhalation. Some upper airway patency must exist to permit egress of gas from the lungs. If gas trapping becomes a problem, passage of a rigid bronchoscope, preferably a pediatric one, transorally to the region of the tracheal introits can sometimes help provide an egress route for gases.

This technique obviously would have limited application in field rescue situations.

5. *Tracheostomy.* Tracheostomy is included only for completeness. Tracheostomy is never an emergency re-oxygenation procedure. Re-oxygenation can always be accomplished using one of the techniques described above.

Even under ideal conditions (good lighting and good assistance) a skilled surgeon may require 15 to 20 minutes to complete a tracheostomy. Trying to reduce the time to a period compatible with escape from serious hypoxic sequelae may very well increase the risk of complications.

While some of the techniques described above do not provide ideal airway control, they do allow emergency re-oxygenation until a definitive method of airway control can be established.

Intrathoracic Impediments to Emergency Oxygenation/Ventilation/Airway Control

Tension Pneumothorax

Patients with closed or penetrating chest trauma must be suspected of having pneumothorax. A simple pneumothorax can be converted rapidly to a tension pneumothorax by IPPV.

As gas is forced from the lung or conducting airway during positive pressure ventilation to the pleural space, the pressure in the affected hemithorax rises. The lung becomes compressed causing increased shunting and hypoxemia. As pressure continues rising, mediastinal shift occurs impairing venous return and cardiac output. As cardiac output falls, the patient displays even more ominous signs of hypoxemia, potentially causing the resuscitist to increase ventilation, thus unknowingly compounding the problem.

Traditional physical signs of pneumothorax (decreased breath sounds, tympany to percussion) are valueless in diagnosing rapidly developing tension pneumothorax in a patient on IPPV. Physical examination may reveal tracheal shift, jugular venous distention, bulging of intercostal spaces and most prominently abdominal distention. This later sign can mislead the resuscitist to think the endotracheal tube has inadvertently entered the esophagus. Abdominal distention is caused by inversion of the diaphragm secondary to the tremendous increase in intrapleural pressure.

If the diagnosis of tension pneumothorax is suspected, the pleural space on at least the affected side and perhaps both sides must be immediately decompressed. A large (12 gauge) intravenous catheter/needle can be inserted into the pleural space on either side at the midclavicle line, second intercostal space, being careful to avoid the neurovascular bundle by sliding the catheter/needle over the superior aspect of the rib. After entering the pleural space the needle is removed leaving the catheter in situ.

Rapid egress of air through the catheter confirms the diagnosis and mandates prompt insertion of pleural drainage tubes.

Cardiac Output Impairment

Any condition substantially impairing cardiac output decreases tissue oxygen delivery. Signs of tissue hypoxia may be seen. At least some physiologic processes impairing cardiac output are also aggravated by respiratory care maneuvers.

For instance, IPPV raises mean intrathoracic pressure. This in turn impairs venous return, thus dropping cardiac output. This phenomenon is exaggerated in the face of hypovolemia, pericardial tamponade and large mediastinal masses. Indeed, transient self-correcting hypotension during IPPV may be one very subtle sign of inadequate blood volume replacement in trauma cases.

Instrumentation of the airway can evoke a massive autonomic nervous system discharge. Most often, sympathetic nervous system signs prevail, but occasionally parasympathetic signs (i.e., bradycardia) are seen.

The propensity for vagotonic bradycardia is increased in extremes of age and pre-existing hypoxia. In these cases atropinization may be helpful prior to airway instrumentation.

Conclusion

The goals of airway control are oxygenation, ventilation and aspiration protection. All are important, but top priority must go to oxygenation.

Airway control methods are divided into cannulating and noncannulating techniques. Mastering noncannulating techniques should be given equal importance with learning cannulating techniques, since the resuscitist must often re-oxygenate using noncannulating methods while cannulation equipment is being prepared or, if indeed, it is not available at all. Airway control, oxygenation and ventilation techniques are ideally learned in the operating room on anesthetized patients under the guidance of experienced anesthesia personnel.

The resuscitist must understand basic respiratory physiology and the interrelationship between respiratory mechanics and cardiovascular function if an optimal approach to the victim of airway compromise is to be planned.

Self-Evaluation Quiz

1. Head tilt is always the first step in securing a patent airway.
   a) True
   b) False
2. IPPV should never be used in partial upper airway obstruction.
   a) True
   b) False
3. A nonrigid catheter is preferred when suctioning liquid material from the mouth since there is less chance of damaging oral mucus membranes than there would be if a rigid pharyngeal tube is used.
   a) True
   b) False
4. Orotracheal intubation is easily and reliably learned by reading and studying diagrams.
   a) True
   b) False
5. Cricothyrotomy is safe, simple and effective and should be taught to the general population.
   a) True
   b) False

Answers on page 289.

Recognition and Initial Management of the Patient With Head Injury

Margaret M. Stevens, R.N., B.S.N.

Objectives

1. To review the abbreviated clinical neurological examination used in identifying neurologic deficits.
2. To review the diagnostic studies utilized for evaluating neurological deficits in the emergency room setting.
3. To present the initial medical management of the patient with neurological disease resulting from trauma.

Introduction

Accidental injury is the leading cause of death in the population between the ages of 2 and 42. Seventy percent of the victims of vehicular accidents have injury to the head [1]. The types of central nervous system (CNS) injuries include mild concussion, major closed head injury, skull fracture, hematomas and spinal trauma (bone, ligamentous and/or nervous damage). The significant injuries require immediate identification and therapy to prevent major complications.

The large number of accident victims are seen initially in the emergency room setting. Rapid identification and treatment of neurologic deficit require capable and experienced personnel in the emergency room (ER). Throughout this discussion, the nursing assessment and medical management are presented to provide the nurse with a current concept of treatment and review of the nursing neurological assessment.

Margaret M. Stevens, R.N., B.S.N., Neurotrauma Nurse Coordinator, Maryland Institute for Emergency Medical Services, Baltimore.

Assessment

Frequently in the community setting, the ER nurse is the first health professional to see the patient. Her initial assessment is crucial, since she then communicates her findings to the physician. A baseline assessment is critical in formulating the nurse's data base for her plan of nursing intervention.

Rapid identification of neurologic deficits requires a preplanned logical approach to assessing the patient. The moment a patient enters the ER doors is not the time to decide how to approach the patient. Time is critical and requires immediate, mature setting of priorities. One must approach the patient with the assumption of multiple trauma until other injuries are ruled out by various diagnostic means.

The nursing assessment of neurologic trauma includes several key neurologic factors: level of consciousness (LOC), pupillary signs, motor signs and abnormalities about the head, face, neck and ears in addition to one's baseline data of the respiratory and cardiovascular systems. It should be noted that the neurosurgeon performs a similar examination with the addition of reflex and cranial nerve evaluation. The presence of respiratory distress and shock always has priority over management of other problems. Without a patent airway and cardiovascular stability, the CNS patient has little chance of surviving to have a mass lesion evacuated.

The LOC, pupil signs and motor activity provide clinical signs of possible mass lesions within the head which become the third priority in management. The nurse determines the patient's LOC by his ability to answer questions and follow commands or the absence of verbal response to questioning. The Glasgow scale is becoming a worldwide method of describing a patient's response so that the complete picture of the patient is described the same way [2]. The terms lethargy, stupor and semicoma are disappearing from the new neurosurgical vocabulary. Currently with the Glasgow scale, the patient is evaluated by his/her verbal response, ability to open the eyes spontaneously and motor movements. The patient with a mass lesion has an altered LOC and may become unresponsive to verbal and noxious stimuli. The patient's orientation to person, place and time can help determine his LOC. Can the individual patient obey simple and complex commands? Does he sleep constantly when left alone? Does he behave as an average, normal individual? Is he aware of the environment but yet does not obey commands, does not seem to understand the spoken word or does not respond by verbal cues or actions? The LOC is determined rapidly at admission time and can be assessed while other components of the exam are done simultaneously. But if tracheal intubation is imminently needed, one must make every effort to evaluate the patient's LOC prior to intubation, and the evaluation must be accomplished rapidly so as not to delay emergency care. The nurse's assessment of LOC is vitally important to the neurosurgeon who may not be able to examine the patient before intubation. Diagnostic studies are also based on the LOC. It should be noted that all forms of severe shock will alter the patient's LOC.

Abnormalities about the face, neck, head and ears also can indicate possible head and neck injuries. Depressions over the skull can indicate depressed skull fracture. Severe head lacerations can produce a shock state from hemorrhage due to the vascularity of the scalp. Bruising behind the ear or Battle's sign suggests possible temporal lobe injuries. Bloody or clear drainage from ears and nose indicates cerebral spinal fluid (CSF) leaks resulting from basilar skull fracture and/or facial fractures.

Pupillary response is another important parameter to be assessed. Equality of the pupils, light reaction and corneal/blink responses are part of the examination. An unconscious patient with unilateral or bilateral dilated fixed pupils requires immediate care to prevent possible brain herniation. One must be aware that facial fractures can lacerate the oculomotor or third cranial nerve as it innervates the eye, thus producing a fixed pupil on the same side. One should also note extraocular movements which indicate brain stem functioning. Assessing extraocular movements involves neck motion, so the ER nurse must know the results of the spinal x-rays before removing any immobilizing devices or turning of the neck.

Motor activities of the patient provide a good clinical picture of the severity and location of injury. Closed head injury frequently produces global trauma in which the entire brain is concussed and contused. The number of primary and secondary sites of injury determine the type of movement of an extremity. Cerebral injury often produces a purposeful (or normal) movement or semipurposeful one in which the patient is unable to localize noxious stimuli. Diencephalic trauma gives a decorticate or a flexor spastic motion. Decerebration or extensor spasticity signals injury within the upper brain stem areas whereas flaccidity is associated with medulla injuries except in the presence of a spinal cord lesion. To determine the type of movement, a maximal pain stimulus should be given. Several areas of the body are appropriate for eliciting a central response to pain — over the eyebrow (after facial fractures are ruled out), muscle mass behind the shoulder, the axillary edge and over the sternum. The stimulus must be painful so that the patient responds at his best.

As motor activity is assessed, one must evaluate the patient for lateralizing signs of weakness, noting whether one side or extremity moves less than the other. The unconscious patient is unable to cooperate with an examiner for assessing fine loss of muscle strength. Maximal pain stimulus allows one to see quickly gross differences in muscle power. Hemiplegia is the most readily observed lack of motor power. Subtle hemiparesis is more difficult to identify on gross examination.

The CNS examination is easily accomplished within one to two minutes and provides several important aspects to the patient's diagnostic studies. Whenever available, any history regarding the patient and the accident from the family or paramedical personnel aids the ER staff in determining neurologic change since the time of impact. Any earlier signs of respiratory or cardiovascular distress at the scene of the accident may help explain the decrease in the LOC.

Throughout the nurse's assessment, one must continually evaluate the patient's status and record it appropriately in a permanent record. Legally and as a means of communication among staff personnel, the recording of neurologic signs is extremely important for optimal patient care.

Diagnostic Studies

After the patient is stabilized and the initial identification of neurologic deficit is made by clinical assessment, a more precise diagnostic means is used to define the type and extent of the injury.

Mechanically controlled ventilation often assists the physician in completing the diagnostic workup without fear of the patient's respiratory status being compromised during the evaluation phase. Ventilation, and specifically hyperventilation, also serves as one of the primary treatments for severe head injury. The use of hyperventilation is an accepted method of providing optimal oxygenation and reduction of cerebral edema.

Angiography is performed to study the brain's vascular system. In the presence of brain trauma, carotid artery punctures are done rather than studies in the vertebral system or brachial and femoral arteries. The neurosurgeon evaluates the angiography for occlusion of cerebral vessels as seen in stroke or shift of normal blood vessels as occurs with space occupying lesions. After withdrawal of the carotid needle, direct pressure over the site is crucial to prevent hematoma formation. One may find it necessary to apply pressure for 10 to 15 minutes with frequent checks after release. Record vital and neurologic signs frequently after angiography. Also observe closely for signs of dye reactions.

Skull x-rays are generally done in the case of cerebral trauma; however, it should be noted that skull films are not an emergency procedure. Care must be taken to see that the patient is stable prior to transport to the x-ray department if a portable machine is unavailable. Skull x-rays for the trauma patient are viewed for fractures, linear or depressed, which can be sources of CSF leaks and shifts in pineal gland which occur when space occupying lesions infringe on the gland.

Computerized axial tomography is rapidly becoming the neurosurgeon's most valuable diagnostic tool. It is a painless procedure for the patient which yields a multitude of data concerning the state of the brain for the physician. The disadvantages of tomography are that the patient must be transported out of the ER for the test and not every hospital is equipped to provide this service. Sedation is, at times, necessary to prevent the patient from moving which alters the quality of the test. Of course, the patient should be accompanied by a nurse or physician to protect the patient's safety during the study.

Electroencephalography (EEG) is not commonly used in the ER setting. It provides a recording of electrical activity of the brain, but the examination is more helpful later in patient evaluation if epilepsy is suspected. The EEG may be done to support clinical evidence of brain death.

Brain scans which involve the use of radioisotope injections can be useful in identifying intracranial hematomas. Again, the patient must be transported to the nuclear medicine division of the x-ray department and not all community hospitals have this service available.

In summary the most common diagnostic studies done in the ER phase are clinical observations, skull and spinal x-rays, and angiography. Where available, the computerized tomography often replaces angiography.

Medical Management

In conjunction with diagnostic workup, several key medications and treatments are initiated. As mentioned previously, hyperventilation by a mechanically controlled method is desirable for providing oxygenation and constriction of the cerebral vessels which decreases the bulk of blood in the brain and reduces the acidosis that occurs with cerebral edema. Ventilation is indicated for any patient who is unable to protect his airway and cough effectively.

Sedation may be necessary to prevent the patient from breathing out of phase or sequence with volume-controlled respirators. Sedation is often contraindicated with the head injured patient because of respiratory depression. Under controlled circumstances, sedatives are effective in maintaining mechanical respiratory control and preventing excessive agitation which can increase cerebral edema. Drugs such as naloxone (Narcan), which is a narcotic antagonist, can remove the narcotics rapidly and allow full evaluation of the patient's clinical picture if questions arise.

A barbiturate-induced coma is under study in several centers in the United States today. Many centers are utilizing specific barbiturate drugs to produce a cerebral-type coma state essentially to allow the brain to rest for several days, thus decreasing activity to minimal levels and reducing cerebral edema. One of the disadvantages of the barbiturate therapy is the prolonged half-life of the drugs which makes evaluation for brain death impossible for several days.

Steroid therapy continues to be a popular method of reducing the brain's inflammatory reactions. A large loading dose of dexamethasone (Decadron) or methylprednisolone (Solu-Medrol) is given initially in the ER, then a reduced maintenance dose is prescribed. Antacids are also prescribed in conjunction with steroids. Any history of ulcerative conditions should be shared with the physician and nursing teams so everyone will be closely observing the patient for potential and/or actual problems.

Diuretics, particularly mannitol, are useful in shrinking brain tissue by their osmotic action. It is a temporary method of reducing cerebral edema. One notices a rapid diuresis within 15 to 30 minutes and an increase in the specific gravity of the urine. Rapid loss of electrolytes may ensue with diuresis.

Intracranial monitoring provides a direct communication with the ventricular system, allowing access to CSF for removal and/or constant monitoring of the pressure within the cranial cavity. Several types of monitoring devices are available. A neurosurgeon may elect to place the catheter several hours to one day after admission. The more severe the brain injury, the greater the necessity for intracranial monitoring. Risks are involved with this form of monitoring. Intracranial devices are very useful in the intensive care setting.

Conclusion

The nurse in the ER plays an important role in the diagnosis and treatment of head injury. Often she is the first to meet and assess the patient. Her findings are communicated to others and priorities are set by initial patient contacts. She protects the rights and safety of the patient as he undergoes testing and treatment. It is the responsibility of the nurse to maintain and continually update her knowledge of neurologic deficit and its current management.

References

1. Accident Facts, 1968-1977. Chicago:National Safety Council, 1977.
2. Langfitt, T.W.: Measuring the outcome from head injuries. J. Neurosurg. 48:673-678, 1978.
3. Gurdjian, E.S. and Gurdjian, E.S.: Acute head injuries. Surg. Gynecol. Obstet. 146:805-820, 1978.

Bibliography

Miller, J.D., Sweet, R.C., Naroyan, R. and Becker, D.P.: Early insults to the injured brain. JAMA 240 (5):439-442, 1978.

Plum, F. and Posner, J. (eds.): The Diagnosis of Stupor and Coma, ed. 2. Philadelphia: Davis, 1972.

Swift, N. and Mabel, R.M.: Manual of Neurological Nursing. Boston: Little, Brown and Company, 1978.

Self-Evaluation Quiz

1. The *most important* aspect(s) of the neurological exam is/are:
   a) Motor movements
   b) Level of consciousness
   c) Pupils
   d) All of these
   e) a and c
2. Decerebration is a flexion movement.
   a) True
   b) False
3. Glasgow scale measures which of the following?
   a) Pupil response
   b) Level of consciousness
   c) Intracranial pressure
   d) Motor responses
   e) All of these
   f) a, b and d
4. Brain scan is an effective diagnostic tool for evaluating head injury.
   a) True
   b) False
5. Computerized tomography is an excellent test because it is:
   a) Inexpensive
   b) Portable
   c) Painless
   d) Performed in the ER with ease
6. Hyperventilation accomplishes which of the following?
   a) Oxygenation
   b) Normal $paCO_2$
   c) Reduces acidosis
   d) Depresses respiration

   e) a and c
   f) a, b and c
7. The EEG is a widely used and effective diagnostic tool with head trauma.
   a) True
   b) False
8. The action of steroid therapy in brain injuries is:
   a) Anti-inflammatory
   b) Diuretic effect
   c) Acidosis reduction
   d) All of those
   e) None of the above

Answers on page 289.

Assessment of Thoracic Trauma

Frank Lewis, Jr., M.D.

Objectives

1. To review the basic management of chest injuries.
2. To recognize the immediate and less life-threatening complications, their diagnosis and treatment.

In the management of thoracic trauma, the principal consideration is that many injuries affecting the chest and heart can lead to rapidly fatal situations. In the emergency room, you must always think of what you can do therapeutically, even when you are uncertain of the diagnosis. Pericardial tamponade and tension pneumothorax are two prime examples and we will examine a several more in this article. I will address this subject from the viewpoint of types of injuries which can be rapidly life-threatening and then discuss a group of injuries that are less life-threatening. I think the biggest trap in dealing with someone who has an obvious thoracic injury is believing that you must have a chest x-ray in order to know exactly what you are dealing with before you begin treating the patient. Realistically, in many cases all that is required, regardless of the disease with which you are dealing, is a chest tube to decompress the tension pneumothorax or to indicate to you the magnitude of the bleeding that is occurring. In severe situations, you may have to decompress the pericardium, if you are dealing with a tamponade. Unless you consider these various things and are ready to deal with them without having all of the diagnostic information, you will lose patients because things move quickly when you have to cope with these types of situations.

Frank Lewis, Jr., M.D., Associate Professor of Surgery; Surgical Director, Intensive Care Unit, San Francisco General Hospital, Calif.; Founding Member, American Trauma Society.

Approximately one quarter of all trauma deaths occur due to thoracic trauma, although many patients die before they get to the hospital. The typical example of this is blunt trauma resulting in aortic arch injuries, transection of the aorta, and massive exsanguination at the scene. Severe blunt trauma may also result in lacerations of the pulmonary hilar structures with massive exsanguination at the scene. Occasionally, very severe blunt trauma results in myocardial rupture. All of these above are irreparable injuries. These patients will die before they reach care. Even if they did reach the hospital, they probably would not be salvageable because the methods for dealing with these injuries are not available.

The conditions with which we really are concerned are those we can treat where a prompt diagnosis and expertise in prompt treatment are critical. Diagnosis is not essential for management in most cases because the initial management demands the placement of a chest tube. In situations where you are quite suspicious that there is a thoracic problem, where the patient presents in respiratory distress, you should not delay diagnostic maneuvers since inserting a chest tube may, in fact, be the major treatment that the patient needs.

In a series of approximately 600 traumatic deaths that we observed, one third of the total could have been prevented by more prompt treatment and diagnosis. This is the background for statements I shall make in this discussion.

There are six conditions that are worthwhile remembering as a diagnostic checklist when you see a patient who is in severe cardiorespiratory distress: (1) a patient who has an open pneumothorax or a sucking chest wound; (2) a patient who has upper airway obstruction; (3) a patient who has a flail chest; (4) a patient who has a tension pneumothorax; (5) massive hemothorax; and (6) cardiac tamponade. All of these conditions can result in rapid death and most are relatively simple to treat. Certainly, the emergency treatment can be carried out quickly in most cases. I will discuss each of these in greater detail to indicate the factors that you need to consider.

Open Pneumothorax

The real problem occurs since the patient's efforts to move air in and out of the lungs are prevented because there is an open communication between the pleural space and the outside air. There is nothing intrinsically wrong with his lung, it is just that the open hole in the thoracic cage prevents him from being able to develop negative intrathoracic pressure and to ventilate normally. The treatment is immediate covering of the communication through the chest wall and, with that, most patients are able to breathe adequately. It is important to understand, in chest physiology, that pneumothorax per se is not the lethal condition. Probably any one of us could tolerate a total pneumothorax on one side with relatively minor respiratory impairment. You might be slightly short of breath and probably would have some pleural pain, but you would not be in severe distress or in extremis, as we are describing in this group of patients. So the problem, when you have an open pneumothorax, is not due to the pneumothorax per se, but it is due to the free movement of air through the chest wall. That fact dictates the immediate treatment, which is to occlude the hole. You can occlude it with anything that is handy. For EMTs out in the field, Vaseline gauze if available is effective, if not, some other dressing to put over it will do. If you are in the emergency room, then you almost certainly will have some method of dressing the wound so that it is airtight. This is usually all that is necessary for immediate treatment.

You then place a chest tube at another site and allow the patient to breathe and close the wound properly at a later time. Immediate treatment simply is to stop the air movement in and out of the chest.

Airway Obstruction

In the emergency situation today, the airway obstruction needs to be dealt with either by removing a foreign body, if that is what is occluding the airway, or by suctioning out secretions. Whenever the patient needs establishment of an airway, we feel very strongly that immediate endotracheal intubation is the procedure to follow. Emergency tracheostomy in the emergency department is a relatively uncommon event today. By and large, the delay necessitated by placing of a tracheostomy is not warranted. The same effect can be attained with an endotracheal tube. Even with severe maxillofacial trauma, a skilled anesthesiologist usually can place an endotracheal tube without difficulty. In any major trauma center, we feel that someone should be available — anesthesiologist or nurse-anesthetist — who is able to do that because establishment of an airway is essential when these patients present. If you have to wait until someone can do an emergency tracheostomy, you will lose several precious minutes that often the patient will not tolerate.

Flail Chest

This is a result of paradoxical movement of a portion of the chest wall when there are multiple rib fractures and usually when ribs are broken at multiple sites. The problem here is analogous in many ways to the open pneumothorax in that the lungs themselves are often not severely damaged. There may be an element of pulmonary contusion in the lung beneath the fractured segment. By and large the respiratory difficulty occurs because the chest wall is unstable, it moves in and out with efforts to breathe, and the development of negative intrathoracic pressure is prevented, which does not allow the patient to move air in and out of his trachea normally. Knowledge of that fact also dictates the treatment, that is, you only need to stabilize the chest wall and it does not have to be stabilized in an outward position; it can be stabilized in an inward position. Simply to prevent the motion of the chest wall in the emergency situation is usually adequate treatment and will relieve the severe respiratory distress that these patients experience. This can be done in the emergency setting by placing a hand against the chest wall to position it, in the ambulance by the use of sand bags or, perhaps the simplest of all, is to turn the patient onto the affected side. If you lay the patient on his side (provided there are no other contraindications to turning him), then his weight lying on the side where the paradox is occurring will prevent that motion and, in addition, the weight of the mediastinum will compress the lower lung which is more likely to be the bad lung and tends to increase the volume of the upper lung. The simplest thing, then, is body position in the emergency setting. When the patient reaches the emergency department, if he is in distress from a flail chest, he should also have immediate intubation and be maintained on positive pressure ventilation in order to achieve internal stabilization of the fractures and to ventilate the lungs adequately.

Massive Hemothorax

Massive hemothorax results from injuries to the aortic arch or to the pulmonary hilum. These types of injuries are usually not salvageable if free rupture has occurred before the patient gets to the hospital. On the other hand, many patients present who will have continuing large rates of blood loss, on the order of 500 to 1000 cc/hr, after presentation to the emergency department. It is essential, in following these patients, that you know the rate of bleeding so that you can replace it on an ongoing basis and keep up with the patient. If you do not know how much he is losing, then you can fall behind and not realize with what you are dealing. Trying to follow the patient by chest x-ray is not an adequate solution. Early placement of chest tubes in any patient who has evidence of intrathoracic blood loss is essential. Close monitoring of the rate of blood loss will let you decide when the patient is going to require surgery, how much blood volume you need to replace, and will provide an ongoing assessment of his status. Generally, the indications for surgery are any patient who continues to bleed in excess of 300 cc/hr over a period of two to three hours or any patient who, on initial placement of the tube, has blood loss in excess of 1 to 1.5 liters. Most of the bleeding that occurs with thoracic injuries is not usually from the lung itself because the lung is a low pressure system and the average pulmonary artery pressure is only about 15 mm Hg, not much above venous pressure. As a result, the patient who continues to bleed is usually doing so from systemic arteries in the chest, that is, the intercostals or the internal mammary. In most patients who are operated on for thoracic bleeding, that is what you find. There are a great majority of patients who have penetrating thoracic trauma who do not require thoracotomy. Approximately 7% to 8% of all patients require surgery, but about 93% do not, because most bleeding that comes from the lung parenchyma will stop.

Cardiac Tamponade

Cardiac tamponade is diagnosed when a patient presents in shock with tightly distended neck veins. Probably, when you are dealing with the diagnosis of the patient in shock, a careful look at the neck veins is the single most important step to take. Always remember to take the time to do this when trying to assess the patient. If you do not see distended neck veins, if they are flat, then you are dealing with a hypovolemic situation. But if the patient has neck veins standing out on the side of his neck like a rope, then you are dealing with either tamponade or a tension pneumothorax. If you have that situation and if the patient is continuing to worsen, try to decompress the tamponade by whatever means is used in your own particular hospital. Most would initially use needle aspiration from the subxyphoid approach. If that is not successful and if the patient worsens, then you need to get him into the operating room immediately, or if the patient arrests in the emergency department, we open the chest immediately and decompress the tamponade there. The specific management in your own particular hospital obviously would depend upon the personnel and facilities you have available. But when dealing with this problem, if the patient is getting steadily worse, there is very little time in which to deal with it and action must be taken very quickly. Needle aspiration will be successful in about 50% of patients as a temporary measure, but it is not the ultimate solution. Ultimately, all of these patients will require decompression.

There are six conditions which are usually somewhat less severe, but also potentially lethal. These represent a second echelon, if you will, of traumatic injuries that you need to consider and treat: (1) rupture or tear of the tracheobronchial tree; (2) pulmonary contusion; (3) rupture of the diaphragm; (4) esophageal perforation; (5) myocardial contusion; and (6) great vessel injury, either by penetrating or nonpenetrating trauma.

Tracheobronchial Tree

Rupture of the tracheobronchial tree is diagnosed by observing the patient who is in respiratory distress with obvious subcutaneous emphysema on initial examination and who has hemoptysis when first examined. The degree of airway obstruction is variable depending upon the nature of the disruption of the tracheobronchial tree. The presence of a tension pneumothorax is variable although the majority of the patients will have some degree of pneumothorax and all will have mediastinal emphysema on chest x-ray. Treatment consists of trying to establish an airway, if possible by getting an endotracheal tube down beyond the region of the tear, so that the patient can be effectively ventilated and will not aspirate blood in the course of spontaneous respiratory efforts. Second, insert a chest tube to evacuate the pneumothorax if the patient has it. Then, operative evaluation by bronchoscopy and immediate operative repair are the modalities of choice.

Pulmonary Contusion

This injury, as discussed earlier, is usually associated with rib fractures. It is nothing more than a bruise of the lung which results most of the time from blunt trauma. For example, it might occur after a high-velocity rifle bullet injury, in which there is severe tissue injury at some distance from the actual bullet track. The treatment is somewhat controversial. In any patient who is hypoxemic as a result of pulmonary contusion, positive pressure ventilation is relatively mandatory until the contusion begins to clear. Diagnosis of contusion rests basically on demonstration of an infiltrate on the first x-ray that you see. Pulmonary contusion is not a lesion that appears three or four days later. It is the patient who has an infiltrate on the first x-ray taken in the emergency department. The degree of the infiltrate will usually progress over the first few days and then begin to clear. Treatment regimens with diuretics, salt-poor albumin and/or steroids are controversial issues and I shall not discuss these here.

Rupture of Diaphragm

This is a particularly subtle diagnosis. You might think it would be very apparent, if you see abdominal viscera in the chest, but it can be extremely subtle and very hard to diagnose. It virtually always occurs on the left side because the liver protects the diaphragm on the right side. The diagnosis is most easily made by having a nasogastric tube in the stomach when you take the chest x-ray because the stomach is the organ that herniates up into the chest through the ruptured diaphragm.

Therefore, if you see the nasogastric tube going down beneath the diaphragm and then curling back up and apparently lying above the diaphragm on the chest film, that will assure you of the diagnosis. This usually does not cause severe respiratory distress although it can, depending upon the other injuries present. Diaphragmatic rupture can be repaired either from above or below the diaphragm, depending upon what other needs the patient has. The condition does need to be repaired promptly, once you have made the diagnosis.

Esophageal Perforation

Most commonly a result of penetrating trauma, this injury rarely occurs with blunt trauma. Depending upon the location, the symptoms will differ. If the perforation is in the cervical area the patient will usually complain of difficulty swallowing and pain on motion of the head. If it is in the thoracic area, the patient will present with fever and chest pain. On x-ray, the patient will have a pneumomediastinum and/or a pleural effusion. The definitive diagnosis is made by having the patient swallow Hypaque and, on x-ray, demonstrate extravasation, or by endoscopy.

Treatment of the cervical perforation is primary repair and drainage. Very rarely, in extremely small perforations, some have advocated expectant treatment, although we do not. Thoracic perforation demands that the patient be explored, the laceration repaired and the chest drained.

Myocardial Contusion

Myocardial contusion is analogous for the myocardium to pulmonary contusion. It is probably a very frequently under-diagnosed condition and it occurs whenever the patient has blunt trauma directly to the anterior chest. In severe cases, myocardial rupture results. These are the patients who never reach the hospital. There are a few cases of late ventricular aneurysm reported but, most of the problems arise from arrhythmias in the immediate peri-injury period. Therefore, if you see a patient who has this sort of injury, an early EKG is mandatory. The most common problems are either atrial arrhythmias or bundle branch block, usually affecting the right more than the left ventricle.

Great Vessel Injury

Penetrating great vessel injuries, if the penetration occurs in the heart in the intrapericardial portion, results in cardiac tamponade. If it is extrapericardial, then hemorrhage into one or the other chest results. We have already discussed those conditions separately.

Blunt trauma to the great vessels most commonly results in transection of the aorta just distal to the origin of the left subclavian. Of all patients who have this injury, about 85% will have free rupture immediately after the injury, but about 15% of patients will survive to reach the hospital. Prompt diagnosis and treatment are mandatory because rupture of the remaining 15% occurs at a declining rate during the first 24 hours. If you do not make the diagnosis and treat the patient promptly and he does rupture into the pleural space the chance of saving him is quite small. The diagnosis is made initially by a history of massive trauma and evidence of mediastinal widening on the chest film. Confirmation of the diagnosis is by aortography.

Summary

Management of chest injuries requires, as with all other injuries, establishment of a patent airway. Be aware of the special problems that can arise with regard to the airway and chest problems. Be sure to evaluate the degree of bleeding in the chest and take measures to control it as quickly as possible. Keep up with replacement while you are evaluating the patient and while diagnostic efforts are proceeding. Be sure that the lungs are satisfactorily expanded by the placement of chest tubes as needed. If the chest wall is unstable, put the patient on positive pressure ventilation for adequate expansion of the lungs and for internal splinting of the fractures. Make sure that the pleural space is adequately drained if hematomas are present there. Remember that the placement of chest tubes requires large-bore #36 or #40 siliconized chest tubes which are the standards that we employ. Finally, debride and close wounds to prevent air leakage into the chest.

Self-Evaluation Quiz

1. In assessing patients with acute trauma to chest one should always consider rapid life-threatening repairable situations. The most common are:
   a) Tension pneumothorax
   b) Myocardial rupture
   c) Pericardial tamponade
   d) Transection of the aorta
   e) a and c
   f) b and d
2. The immediate problems that also should be considered that may be rapidly life-threatening are:
   a) Sucking chest wounds
   b) Massive hemothorax
   c) Upper airway obstruction
   d) All of the above
   e) None of the above
3. The immediate treatment of an open pneumothorax is:
   a) Start a large bore intravenous catheter
   b) Place the patient on oxygen
   c) Close the hole with vaseline gauze
   d) a, b and c
   e) None of the above
4. Immediate emergency outpatient treatment of flail chest is:
   a) To stabilize the chest wall
   b) To stabilize the chest wall in an outward position
   c) Endotracheal intubation at all times
   d) Intubation on negative pressure ventilation
   e) None of the above
5. Methods of treating flail chest is(are):
   a) Turn the patient opposite to the affected side
   b) Turn patient onto the affected side
   c) Immediate intubation on positive pressure ventilator if stabilization fails
   d) a and c
   e) b and c
6. The indications for surgery in patients with massive hemothorax are:
   a) When patients bleed in excess of 300 ml/hr
   b) On tube placement 50 ml of blood obtained

c) When chest tube is placed 2 liters of blood is obtained
d) When blood pressure is low
e) a and c
f) b and d

7. The incidence of patients requiring chest tube placement *and* thoracotomy is:
   a) 7%
   b) 20%
   c) 40%
   d) 60%
   e) 80%
8. Cardiac tamponade is best diagnosed:
   a) By chest x-ray
   b) When neck veins are flat
   c) When a patient presents in shock with tightly distended neck veins
   d) By electrocardiogram
   e) All of the above

Answers on page 289.

Diagnosis and Treatment of Acute Ocular Trauma

L. Morgan Hale, M.D., F.A.C.S.

Objectives

Ocular trauma is a leading cause of blindness in the United States. The purpose of this presentation is to review the most common forms of ocular trauma with special emphasis on clinical diagnosis and proper management.

Introduction

Following ocular trauma, the ultimate preservation of a visually functioning eye may depend as much upon the prompt assessment of the injury and initial care by emergency personnel as upon the ophthalmologist who provides follow-up care. Indeed, the first person to treat the injured eye may be the most important person involved in the determination of the final visual result.

Forms of ocular trauma include blunt trauma (contusions), abrasions, lacerations, foreign bodies, thermal, chemical and radiant energy injuries.

Eyelid Contusions

The loose areolar tissue of the outer third of the eyelids has a rich blood supply. Contusions commonly cause hemorrhage into the eyelids, the common "black eye" (Figs. 1A and 2). The hemorrhage may be in the form of a localized hematoma or, more commonly, a diffuse ecchymosis. The hemorrhage may

---

L. Morgan Hale, M.D., F.A.C.S., Clinical Associate Professor of Ophthalmology, The University of North Carolina School of Medicine, Chapel Hill.

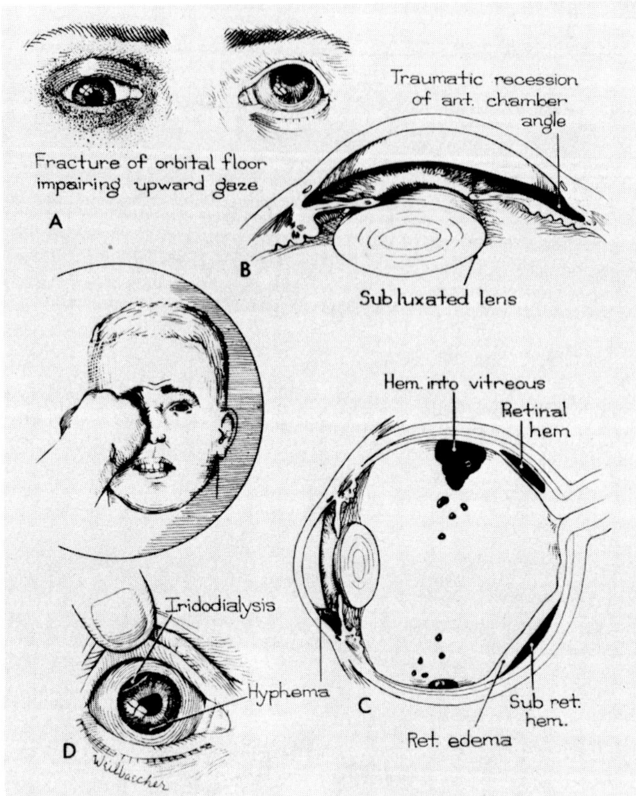

FIG. 1. Ocular complications following contusion injuries.

dissect under the bridge of the nose to the opposite eyelids or down into the cheek giving the false impression of more extensive damage. However, the presence of any eyelid ecchymosis indicates trauma severe enough to potentially damage the orbital bones or the globe. Frequently, eyelid ecchymoses are associated with subconjunctival hemorrhages and, less commonly, orbital hematomas (Fig. 2). Eyelid ecchymosis may be associated with orbital roof fractures, blow-out fractures of the orbital floor or basilar skull fractures.

The globe must be carefully examined after any contusion injury to rule out occult intraocular damage (Fig. 1). On occasion, the ecchymosis may be so large that eyelid retractors are required in order to open the eyelids well enough to

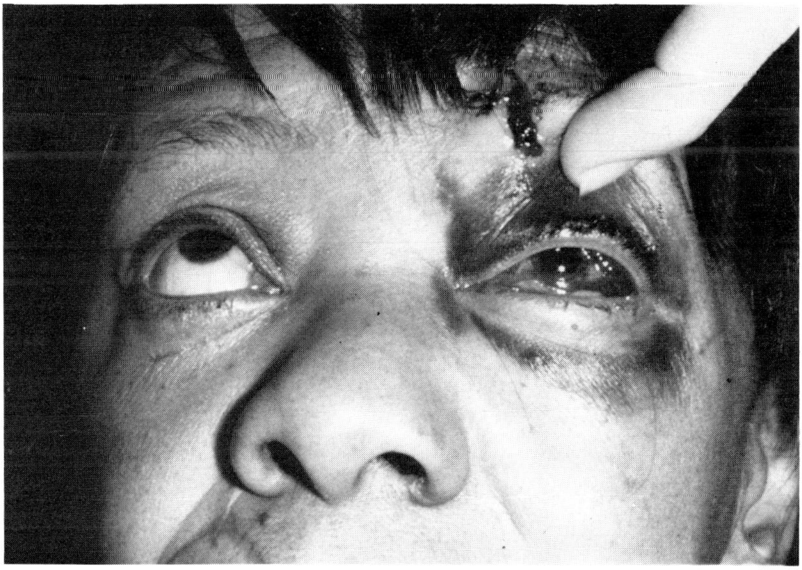

FIG. 2. Blow-out fracture of left orbit showing eyelid ecchymosis, subconjunctival hemorrhage, enophthalmos and limitation of upper gaze.

examine the globe. Care must be taken to not put undue pressure on the eyelids since there may be an unsuspected perforation of the globe.

Uncomplicated ecchymoses generally clear within a 10- to 14-day period, and the only treatments required are cold compresses to reduce edema and hemorrhage, followed by warm compresses to aid blood absorption.

Conjunctival Contusions

Frequently, subconjunctival hemorrhages are associated with eyelid contusions (Fig. 2). They may also occur after strangulation, gagging or vomiting. The common spontaneous subconjunctival hemorrhage seen in older patients is usually due to mild ocular trauma or straining. Anatomically, subconjunctival hemorrhages cannot spread past the corneal limbus, thus visual acuity is never impaired. If vision is decreased, careful evaluation must be made of the entire globe to rule out intraocular damage (Fig. 1). Like eyelid ecchymoses, subconjunctival hemorrhages clear within 10 to 14 days. No treatment is indicated unless the hemorrhage is massive enough to cause conjunctival prolapse. This requires instillation of lubricating ointments until the prolapse subsides.

A benign appearing subconjunctival hemorrhage may mask a penetrating or lacerating injury of the underlying sclera. Therefore, careful examination of the hemorrhagic area is required to rule out occult injuries.

Orbital Bone Fractures

The globe sits in the orbit protected by periorbital fat and orbital bones (Fig. 3C). Blunt trauma compresses the orbital contents, and if the pressure is great enough, the globe may rupture or an orbital bone fracture may occur. Trauma severe enough to cause orbital fractures is frequently associated with eyelid ecchymoses, subconjunctival hemorrhage, diplopia, intraocular damage, enophthalmos or proptosis from orbital hemorrhage or edema.

The thin medial wall of the orbit separates the orbital contents from the ethmoid sinuses. Clinically, a fracture into

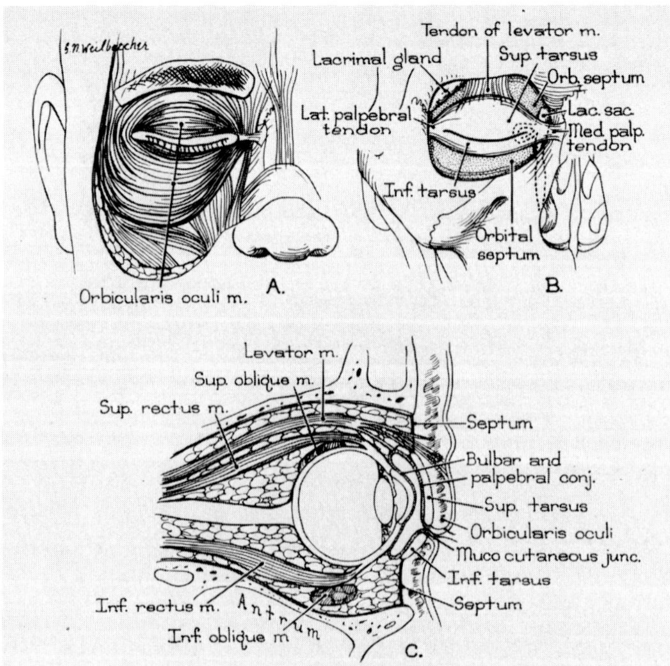

FIG. 3. Anatomy of the orbit and eyelids.

the ethmoids may be associated with epistaxis and emphysema (air crepitus) into the upper eyelid and, less commonly, beneath the conjunctiva. A trapped medial rectus muscle will cause limitation of abduction of the globe. If an associated sinusitis is present, the possibility of a secondary bacterial orbital cellulitis exists. Radiologic evidence of an ethmoid fracture indicates the need for prophylactic systemic antibiotics.

The most common orbital fracture occurs through the floor of the orbit into the underlying maxillary sinus where prolapsed inferior rectus and oblique muscles and orbital fat are trapped by the bony fragments (Figs. 1A and 2). The patient is unable to fully elevate the injured eye as well as the uninjured eye. Frequently, anesthesia of the lower eyelid and side of the nose is present due to damage to the second division of the fifth cranial nerve which runs along the floor of the orbit. In addition to infraorbital facial anesthesia and limitation of upward gaze, enophthalmos, eyelid ecchymosis and subconjunctival hemorrhage may be present. Facial x-rays (Waters view) may show the typical "hanging drop of fat" protruding into the maxillary sinus. However, a traumatic submucosal hematoma or cyst in the maxillary sinus may mimic the "hanging fat" sign. Since orbital hemorrhage and edema themselves may cause limitation of ocular gaze, a misinterpreted maxillary sinus hematoma may lead to a mistaken diagnosis of a blow-out fracture of the orbit. Therefore, forced ductions under topical anesthesia and orbital tomograms or CT scan are needed to verify the diagnosis of an orbital floor fracture.

Blow-out fractures generally do not require immediate surgical repair. However, frequently there is associated intraocular injury following a blow severe enough to cause a blow-out fracture. Therefore, the globe must be examined carefully for associated injuries. If the globe does not require immediate surgical care, the blow-out fracture may be repaired at a later date, if necessary. The decision to surgically repair a blow-out fracture depends primarily upon whether significant diplopia persists or enophthalmos is present.

Iris Trauma

Any form of ocular trauma may irritate the iris enough to cause traumatic iritis. Typically, the patient will complain of a mild to severe aching photophobic eye. Photophobia is due to irritation of the iris sphincter muscle which contracts in a painful, cramplike fashion, especially when exposed to bright light. Clinically, conjunctival and episcleral blood vessels around the limbus are dilated — the typical circumcorneal flush. The pupil is miotic due to sphincter muscle spasm. Slit lamp examination of the aqueous shows inflammatory cells and protein from leaking iris and ciliary body blood vessels.

The time-honored treatment of iritis is dilation of the pupil with cycloplegics such as short-acting homatropine or longer-acting atropine. Mydriasis promptly relieves sphincter muscle spasm and reduces the exudation of protein and inflammatory cells into the anterior chamber. Topical corticosteroids further reduce iris inflammation after blunt trauma, but must *never* be used after an abrasion or foreign body injury due to the risk of secondary bacterial, fungal and viral infection. As a general rule, no ophthalmic corticosteroids, whether alone or combined with antibiotics, should ever be used without ophthalmology consultation.

In some cases following blunt trauma, the pupil may be irregularly dilated rather than miotic, due to rupture of the iris sphincter muscle. This allows the unopposed iris dilator muscle to dilate a segment of the pupil. At other times, the iris root may be torn from its insertion into the sclera (Fig. 4). This iridodialysis may persist with a pupil in the shape of a capital D (Fig. 1D). Any pupil irregularity following blunt trauma indicates the possibility of associated intraocular damage and the globe must be carefully examined.

Anterior Chamber Hemorrhage (Hyphema)

Blunt trauma frequently causes rupture of an iris blood vessel and the resultant hemorrhage into the anterior chamber is a hyphema (Figs. 1C, 1D and 4). In addition to bleeding from a ruptured iris vessel, the iris sphincter may be torn or an iridodialysis may be present (Figs. 1D and 4). All injured eyes should be examined with a slit lamp, since some hyphemas may be microscopic and not grossly visible. Microscopic hyphemas, with red blood cells in suspension in the aqueous, should be treated with the same concern as grossly visible hyphemas. Hyphemas may partially or totally fill the anterior chamber and

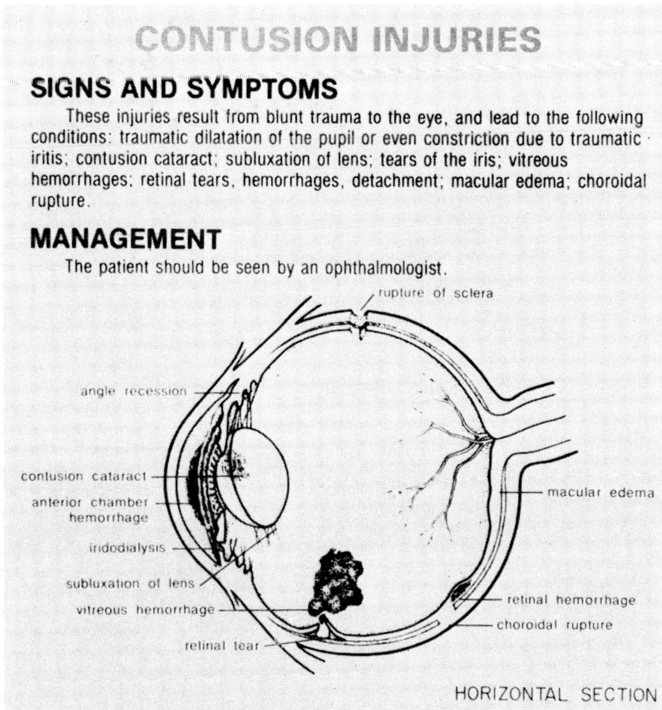

FIG. 4. Contusion injuries.

displace enough aqueous to cause secondary glaucoma. Secondary glaucoma must be treated medically with osmotic agents such as oral acetazolamide and topical epinephrine drops. If the elevated pressure persists for several days despite maximum medical therapy and the hyphema shows no evidence of absorption, paracentesis of the anterior chamber may be required to evacuate the blood. In most cases, hyphemas spontaneously absorb within three to five days. However, as many as 20% may spontaneously rebleed between the third and fifth posttrauma day. Therefore, these eyes must be followed closely, for the second hemorrhage may be more severe than the original. This increases the chance of complications such as secondary glaucoma or blood staining of the cornea. Hyphemas are frequently associated with traumatic recession of the anterior chamber angle and damage to the trabecular meshwork (Figs. 1B and 4). This can only be detected by slit lamp examination with a gonioprism contact lens. The presence of angle recession increases the future chance of secondary glaucoma; therefore, a yearly intraocular pressure check is indicated.

Crystalline Lens Trauma

The crystalline lens is suspended by zonules from the ciliary body. Following blunt trauma, rupture of the suspensory zonules may allow partial or complete dislocation of the lens posteriorly into the vitreous or anteriorly into the pupil or anterior chamber (Figs. 1B and 4). Rapid eye movements may show quivering of the iris (iridodenesis) if the lens is no longer in contact with the posterior iris. Posterior dislocation of the lens into the vitreous causes deepening of the anterior chamber and late ocular inflammation. Anterior dislocation of the lens into the pupil may block the flow of aqueous into the anterior chamber and lead to pupillary block glaucoma. On occasion, the lens may prolapse through the pupil into the anterior chamber where it causes secondary glaucoma. Anteriorly dislocated lenses may require surgical removal in order to restore normal aqueous flow and alleviate secondary glaucoma. However, glaucoma may persist if there is associated trabecular damage.

Blunt trauma may cause anterior or posterior cortical cataracts although these are seldom obvious at the time of injury (Fig. 4). Careful slit lamp examination, with the pupil dilated, may detect early cataract changes which can progress rapidly to cause significant visual impairment.

Contusions may press the iris forcibly against the anterior lens capsule leaving a circular ring of pigment called a Vossius ring. This does not progress nor cause visual difficulty.

Penetrating lens injuries lead to opacification of lens fibers. If the laceration is small, it may be sealed off by fibrous metaplasia and the traumatic cataract may remain localized. More commonly, however, there is immediate opacification and flocculation of lens material with subsequent loss of visual acuity. Slit lamp examination through a well-dilated pupil allows best evaluation of the lens injury. Penetrating lens injuries may allow leakage of lens protein into the anterior chamber causing secondary iritis and phacolytic glaucoma. Phacolytic glaucoma is due to occlusion of the trabecular meshwork in the anterior chamber with lens protein laden macrophages.

Vitreous, Retina and Choroid Trauma

The vitreous body is located behind the iris and lens and in front of the retina. The vitreous is a jell-like substance which has fine microscopic attachments to the peripheral and peripapillary retina. Ocular trauma may cause a tear in retinal, choroidal or ciliary body blood vessels leading to hemorrhage into the retina or the vitreous (Figs. 1C and 4). Vitreous hemorrhages are often associated with decreased visual acuity. The retina must be carefully examined, for these hemorrhages may be due to retinal tears which may cause subsequent retinal detachments (Fig. 4). Many retinal tears are in the periphery of the retina where they can be detected only after full dilation of the pupil and examination with an indirect ophthalmoscope. Unless the patient notes decreased vision, flashes of light from vitreous tugging on the retina (photopsia) or vitreous floaters or opacities, the retinal tear may not be apparent until a significant visual field defect is present from a retinal detachment. Therefore, any eye that sustains blunt trauma, with or without vitreous hemorrhage, should be dilated and examined by an ophthalmologist for a peripheral retinal tear.

The presence of a vitreous hemorrhage after a head injury is at times associated with a subdural hematoma. Thus, any patient with a head injury and vitreous hemorrhage should be observed carefully for other neurological signs.

The anatomical posterior pole of the eye is the macular and the central fovea, which are used for central vision. Force from an anterior ocular contusion is transmitted to the back of the globe with resultant macular edema (Berlin's edema, commotio retinae) and/or macular hemorrhage (Figs. 1C and 4). This usually immediately reduces central visual acuity and may lead to permanent visual loss due to macular scarring or atrophic macular holes. Any eye that does not have equally good vision compared to the uninjured eye should be suspected of having a contusion injury of the macular area, and ophthalmology consultation is indicated.

The choroid is the highly vascular layer of the globe which separates the inner retina from the outer sclera. Ocular contusions may cause a posterior pole choroidal rupture which initially may appear to be a subretinal hemorrhage (Fig. 4). This gradually heals to form a dark hypertrophic posterior pole scar. If the overlying retina is also involved, it is referred to as chorioretinitis sclopetaria.

Optic Nerve Trauma

The optic nerve may be injured by contusions, especially to the eyebrow area, or by penetrating missiles. The optic nerve is relatively immobile in the posterior orbit and optic canal. Thus, it is vulnerable to contusion effects such as optic nerve edema, ischemia and optic nerve sheath hemorrhages. Fractures of the optic canal frequently result in decreased visual acuity and visual field defects. Avulsions of the optic nerve, causing unilateral blindness, are not too common and are usually associated with fractures of the lateral orbital wall. Initially, the optic disc may appear normal or edematous following contusions or penetrating injuries, but late optic atrophy generally ensues.

Ocular Foreign Bodies

Ocular foreign bodies may be external, intraocular or intraorbital.

Conjunctival foreign bodies are generally easily detected. Usually they are not particularly painful and the patient may complain only of slight irritation or a red eye. If the foreign body is located on or in the conjunctiva, it will move freely when a cotton-tipped applicator moves the loosely connected adjacent conjunctiva over the sclera. However, if the foreign body does not move as the adjacent conjunctiva is moved, this may indicate penetration into the underlying sclera, and removal may result in prolapse of intraocular tissue (Fig. 5). These immobile conjunctival foreign bodies should be evaluated by slit lamp examination by an ophthalmologist prior to their removal.

Most conjunctival foreign bodies are removed easily with a cotton-tipped applicator after instillation of topical anesthetics. Occasionally, however, the foreign body must be removed with small forceps or surgically excised. Following the removal of a

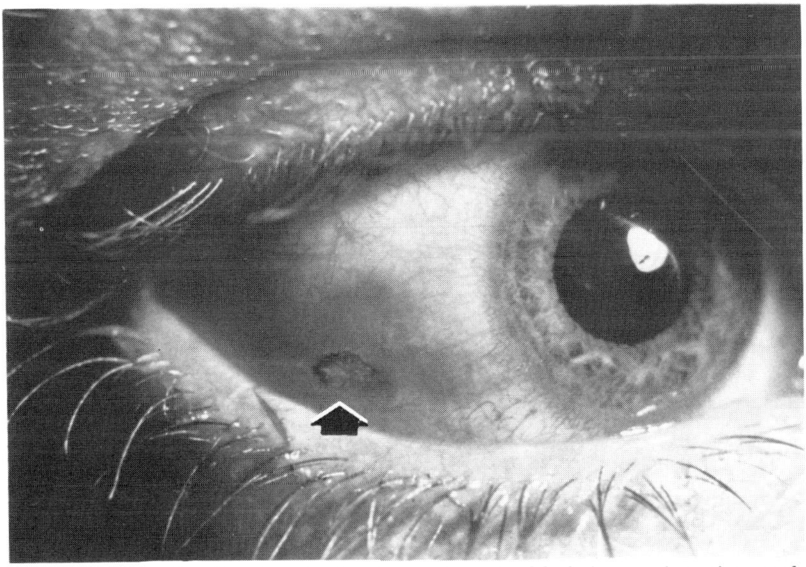

FIG. 5. Metallic foreign body (*arrow*) embedded in conjunctiva and underlying sclera. Subconjunctival hemorrhage masks scleral penetration site.

conjunctival foreign body, prophylactic broad-spectrum antibiotic eye drops, such as sulfacetamide, should be used until the eye is clear of infection. As with any other ocular injury, no corticosteroids should be used without ophthalmology consultation.

Frequently, a small foreign body will be trapped under the eyelid on the tarsal conjunctiva where it abrades the upper cornea with each blink. Clinically, the superior cornea will stain with fluorescein. Tarsal foreign bodies may be seen by everting the upper eyelid, and they are easily removed with a cotton-tipped applicator without topical anesthesia. Since the cornea is usually abraded by the tarsal foreign body, prophylactic antibiotic eye drops should be instilled until the cornea no longer stains. Any associated iritis should be treated with cycloplegics; however, no corticosteroids should be used as long as the cornea stains with fluorescein.

Corneal foreign bodies are common ocular injuries. Many are metallic and firmly embedded in the soft corneal epithelium. If allowed to remain on the cornea for more than 24 hours, ferrous metallic foreign bodies begin to rust and this makes removal more difficult (Fig. 6). After application of topical anesthesia, corneal foreign bodies may be irrigated, removed with a cotton-tipped applicator, or more commonly removed with a small spud or hypodermic needle. Any residual rust ring must be carefully dissected out of the foreign body site in order to assure proper healing. No foreign body should be removed with a needle unless one has adequate magnification and illumination due to the risk of anterior chamber penetration. The cornea should be patched daily with broad-spectrum antibiotics to insure against secondary infection. Absolutely no corticosteroids should be used due to the risk of secondary infections. Secondary iritis should be treated with cycloplegics.

The possibility of a perforating intraocular foreign body should always be suspected (Fig. 7). The perforation site may be small and appear to be nothing more than a subconjunctival hemorrhage. If the patient gives a history of striking metal upon metal and no foreign body can be found on the external surface of the eye, an x-ray of the orbit should be obtained to rule out an intraocular foreign body.

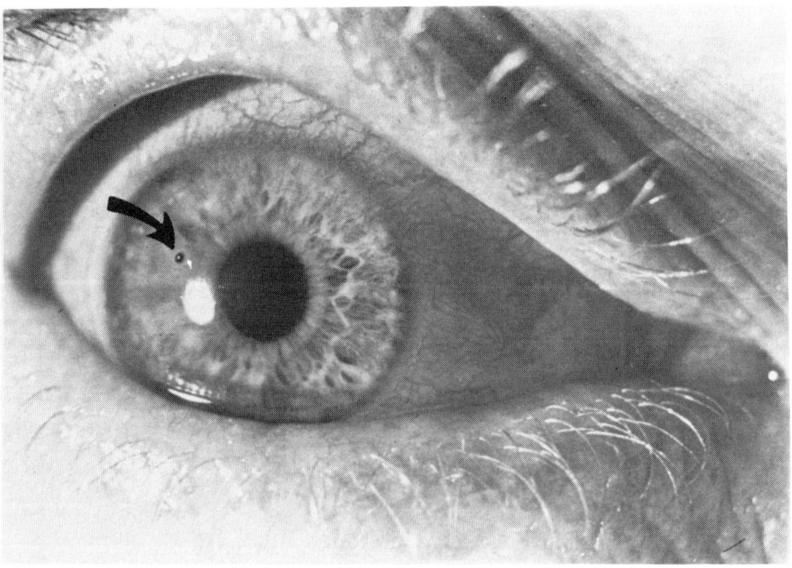

FIG. 6. Rusting metallic corneal foreign body (*arrow*) with secondary iritis (circumcorneal flush and slightly miotic pupil).

INTRAOCULAR FOREIGN BODY

SIGNS AND SYMPTOMS

1. Suspect an intraocular foreign body when a patient complains of sudden sharp pain in the eye, and blurry vision.
2. Inspect the cornea, conjunctiva, iris, and anterior surface of the lens carefully for small lacerations or other possible sites of entry.

MANAGEMENT

Patch eye with sterile dressing and eye shield and refer patient to ophthalmologist.

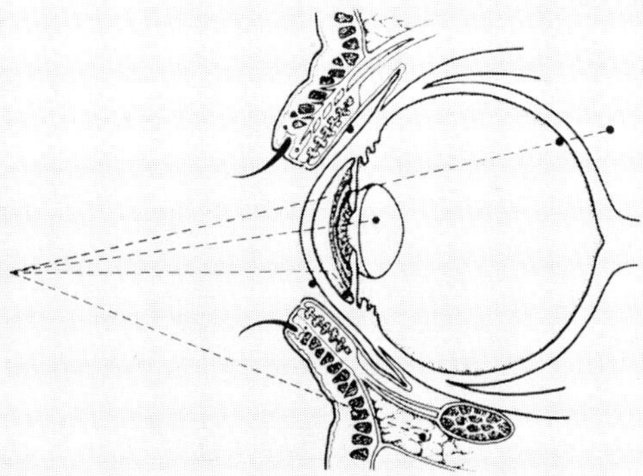

FIGURE 7.

The decision whether to remove an intraocular foreign body depends upon the nature of the foreign body, its known effect on the globe, its magnetic properties, its surgical accessibility and the anticipated surgical trauma involved in its removal. Inert foreign bodies such as glass or stone cause very little ocular inflammation after the initial damage. Removal of inert foreign bodies is determined by their accessibility at the time of closure of the penetration site.

Metallic foreign bodies, depending upon their composition, may be extremely damaging to the globe, both immediately and subsequently. Metals with a high ferrous content may cause siderosis bulbi, a disastrous late inflammation of the globe. The inflammation occurs due to intracellular deposition of ferrous material in the cornea, iris, lens and retina. Early removal of a known metallic foreign body with high ferrous content is indicated.

Copper, brass and bronze foreign bodies produce degeneration of the globe called chalcosis. Copper foreign bodies may produce immediate mild or severe inflammation as well as long-term degeneration. In children, an all-too-often seen copper intraocular foreign body is the useless lethal BB. Fortunately, these destructive "toys" have a magnetic core within the nonmetallic copper casing which facilitates their surgical removal.

Missile-type foreign bodies frequently cause double perforations and finally lodge outside the globe in the orbit (Fig. 7). Globes with double perforations generally have a poor prognosis. Prior to surgical exploration, localization x-rays will help determine whether the foreign body is intraocular or intraorbital. If possible, a similar piece of metal, if it can be obtained, should be examined to determine its magnetic properties.

The immediate treatment of a suspected perforating foreign body injury is a light eye patch and a protective eye shield. The patient should be kept as quiet as possible to avoid straining which could lead to tissue prolapse. No ointment should be applied to the eye since it must be removed at the time of surgical repair and may also cause intraocular inflammation. Immediate ophthalmology consultation is indicated.

Corneal Abrasions

Corneal abrasions are frequent ocular injuries resulting from objects striking the epithelial surface of the cornea or from overwearing contact lenses. Most are superficial and do not extend beneath the five-cell-thick corneal epithelial surface. However, they are painful and may be associated with secondary iritis. Fingernail and pine needle abrasions seem to cause more pain and inflammation than similar sized abrasions from other causes, probably due to keratin and pine resin irritation.

Corneal abrasions should be suspected when the patient complains of pain on blinking. At times, the pain may be so severe that topical anesthetics are required to relieve the associated blepharospasm. Corneal abrasions may be confirmed by applying sterile fluorescein to the injured cornea. Abrasions will stain light green compared to the remainder of the uninjured cornea (Fig. 8). Even small abrasions may be seen

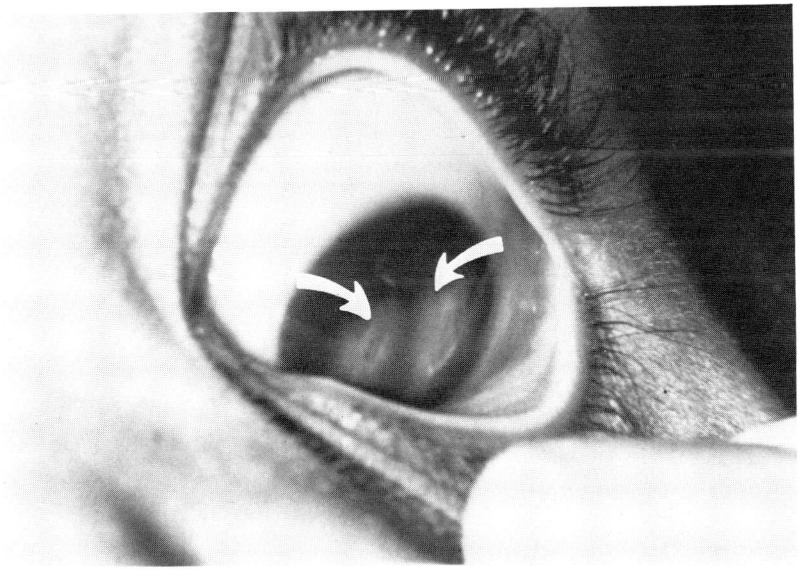

FIG. 8. Fluorescein staining corneal abrasions (*arrows*).

with good magnification; however, slit lamp examination is best for detecting minor corneal abrasions and secondary iritis. If the superior cornea stains, the upper eyelid must be everted since a tarsal foreign body may be present.

Uncomplicated superficial epithelial corneal abrasions heal without permanent scarring or loss of vision. However, if Bowman's membrane or the deeper corneal stroma are involved, by either the original injury or secondary infection, permanent scarring may occur. No corticosteroids should be applied to the injured cornea due to the risk of secondary infection.

The treatment of a corneal abrasion is application of a topical broad-spectrum antibiotic, such as sulfacetamide, and dilation of the pupil with cycloplegics if iritis is present. A firm eye patch to splint the eyelid is helpful in reducing discomfort. However, the abrasion will heal as quickly with or without a patch. Mild analgesics may be needed for pain during the first 24 hours. The patient should not be given topical anesthetics, because these reduce epithelial migration and regeneration and retard corneal healing.

If the abrasion is due to contact lens wear, the lens should not be worn again until the corneal epithelium has healed well and matured. During this healing period, the contact lens should be checked for warpage.

Days, weeks or months after a corneal abrasion the patient may awaken with sharp pain and lacrimation in the injured eye. Slit lamp examination will reveal a recurrent staining defect at the site of the original injury. This recurrent corneal erosion may be due to faulty attachment of the healing epithelial cells to the underlying basement membrane or it may be due to a "fingerprint" dystrophy of the cornea. Recurrent corneal erosions following abrasions should be evaluated by an ophthalmologist. Frequently, lubricating ointment is required at bedtime for many months in order to minimize adhesions between the eyelid and the loose corneal epithelium.

Eyelid Lacerations

The eyelids are divided into overlying epithelium, subcutaneous tissue, orbicularis muscle fibers, tarsus and conjunctiva (Fig. 3). The orbital septum connects the margins of the upper and lower tarsi to the orbital rim and acts as an orbital "fire wall" (Fig. 3). It prevents superficial eyelid infections, such as styes, from penetrating into the orbit and also prevents the anterior prolapse of orbital fat. Superficial horizontal lacerations not involving the eyelid margin or orbital septum may be closed with small interrupted sutures and dressed with antibiotic ointment. However, deeper lacerations may involve the orbital septum or globe. Thus, any eyelid laceration, no matter how superficial it appears, must be carefully inspected for prolapsed orbital fat. The presence of orbital fat indicates laceration of the orbital septum and this increases the likelihood of underlying globe damage (Fig. 9). An ophthalmology consultation is indicated.

The upper and lower eyelids unite medially and laterally to form common palpebral (canthal) tendons which insert into the medial and lateral orbital rims and anchor the eyelids in their normal horizontal position (Fig. 3B). Lacerations in the outer canthal area may sever the insertion of the lateral palpebral tendon. Usually the lateral palpebral tendon is easily palpated just inside the orbital rim if eyelid edema is not present. If the severed tendon is not resutured to the orbital rim, the eyelids

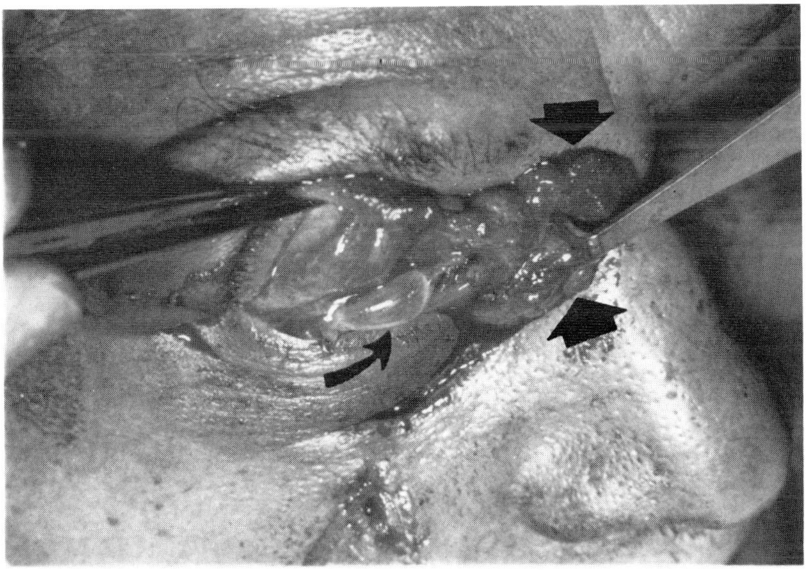

FIG. 9. Laceration of orbital septum with prolapse of orbital fat (*large arrows*) and prolapse of intraocular contents (*small curved arrow*) from underlying globe laceration.

may have an undesirable cosmetic appearance following repair of the laceration.

Medially, in the upper and lower eyelids, the lacrimal puncta and caniliculi drain into the tear sac which is located in the lacrimal fossa of the nasal bone (Figs. 3B and 10). A medial eyelid laceration must be carefully examined to assure that the lacrimal structures are not involved. If the caniliculis is severed it must be repaired with a "splint" which joins the severed ends. If the ends are not properly reunited, annoying epiphora may result from tears not properly draining from the lacrimal lake into the tear sac. Ophthalmology consultation is indicated for any medial canthal laceration involving the lacrimal structures.

The tendon of the levator muscle which raises the upper eyelid inserts primarily in the upper tarsus (Fig. 3B). Deep horizontal lacerations of the upper eyelid may sever the attachment of the levator to the upper tarsus (Fig. 10). The levator tendon must be resutured to the tarsus in order to avoid permanent traumatic ptosis. Levator function must be evaluated prior to repair of the upper eyelid laceration. If the laceration is deep enough to sever the levator tendon, it is potentially deep enough to lacerate the extraocular muscles or globe, and ophthalmology consultation is indicated.

Vertical eyelid lacerations involving the lid margin present special problems in surgical repair because of their tendency to "notch" (Fig. 10). Notching, which is more common in the upper eyelid, is caused by the horizontal pull of the orbicularis muscle fibers against the vertical laceration line (Fig. 3A). It may be avoided by meticulous layer by layer approximation of eyelid tissue with fine interrupted sutures. Ophthalmology consultation is indicated for any eyelid margin laceration because frequently the underlying globe is also involved.

It is unusual to actually lose eyelid tissue even in severe lacerations. With care, eyelid lacerations may be reapproximated like a jigsaw puzzle with generally good cosmetic results. Since the eyelid has a rich blood supply, infection is uncommon. Therefore, it is unnecessary to sacrifice tissue during

EYELID LACERATIONS

Minor horizontal lacerations of the eyelids not involving the eyelid margin can be repaired by using fine sutures. The following lacerations should be evaluated by a qualified specialist:

1. Deep lacerations across the upper eyelid which may involve the levator muscle.
2. Lacerations of the eyelid margin.
3. Medial canthal lacerations which may involve the canaliculi.

COMPLICATIONS DUE TO INADEQUATE REPAIR

1. Ptosis.
2. Eyelid notching.
3. Obstruction of the lacrimal drainage system.
4. Entropion and ectropion.

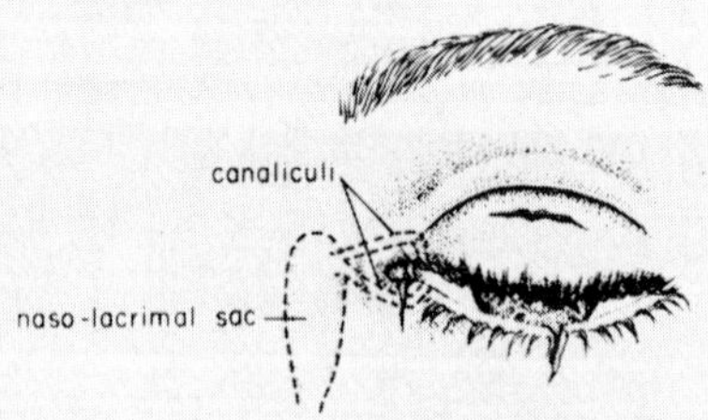

FIGURE 10.

debridement. While most eyelid lacerations heal with good cosmetic results, extensive vertical lacerations may result in ectropion from scar tissue contraction. This is more common in patients who have a tendency to heal with "keloid" type scars. When it is anticipated a large laceration may result in extensive vertical contraction, a tarsorrhaphy should be considered. This will vertically anchor the upper and lower eyelids together and hold them in normal position until the scar tissue has ceased contracting.

Animal bites in the eyelid area are a cause for great concern due to the possibility of anaerobic and aerobic infection and rabies. Frequently, these injuries occur in children as a result of dog bites. The wound should be thoroughly debrided and ophthalmology consultation should be obtained prior to suturing the wound. Some surgeons believe that healing should be by secondary intention whereas others feel suturing is indicated. Careful examination of the underlying globe is necessary in order to rule out associated ocular damage. Systemic antibiotics are usually indicated as well as consideration of antirabies serum.

Conjunctival Lacerations

Small lacerations of the conjunctiva generally do not require suturing. However, the possibility of extraocular muscle involvement or a deeper scleral injury must always be considered. Subconjunctival hemorrhages may obscure vitreous, uveal or retinal prolapse; therefore, the laceration site must be carefully examined under topical or local anesthesia for hidden scleral damage. Uncomplicated conjunctival lacerations generally heal within a few days and the only treatment required is the application of broad-spectrum antibiotics.

Corneal and Scleral Lacerations

Most corneal and anterior scleral lacerations are clinically apparent unless hidden by the eyelid or obscured by an overlying subconjunctival hemorrhage (Fig. 11). Posterior lacerations may be more difficult to recognize since the laceration site is not visible. Both anterior and posterior lacerations may cause shallow or flat anterior chambers,

RUPTURED GLOBE

SIGNS AND SYMPTOMS

1. Decrease in visual acuity to hand movements or light projection.

2. Lowered intraocular pressure (soft eye).

3. Flat or shallow anterior chamber (iris up against or very close to cornea) and hyphema (blood inside eye).

4. If rupture is anterior, ocular contents may be visibly extruding.

MANAGEMENT

1. Eye should be protected with sterile dressing and eye shield. Ointment should **not** be used. Avoid pressure on the globe.

2. Patient is warned not to squeeze his eye shut. Binocular patching advisable to prevent eye movements.

3. Do not attempt to remove any blood clots, foreign bodies, or tissue from the eye.

4. An analgesic and sedative may be required while waiting for the ophthalmologist.

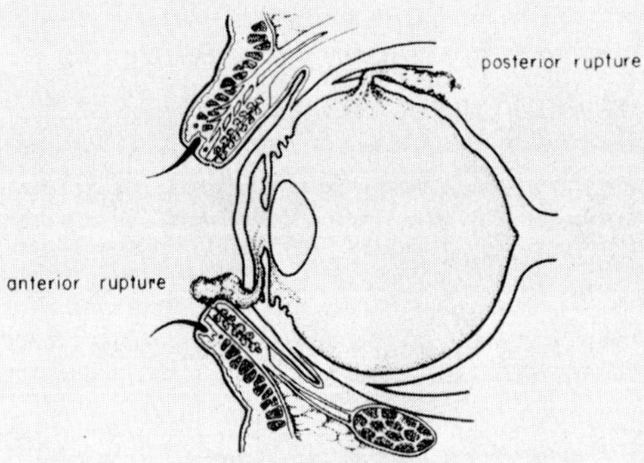

FIGURE 11.

prolapsed intraocular contents, decreased visual acuity and low intraocular tension.

The initial treatment of a penetrating injury to the globe is conservative in order to prevent further loss of intraocular contents. A sterile eye patch should be applied and the patient kept quiet and prone. No pressure should be applied to the eye. If antibiotics must be applied, they should be in drop rather than ointment form. Surgical repair as quickly as possible is indicated to prevent further loss of intraocular tissue and prevent secondary endophthalmitis.

Thermal Burns

Most flash burns primarily involve the eyelids. The underlying globe is generally spared due to the rapid protective blink and Bell's reflex. First degree burns of the eyelids cause mild to moderate discomfort, edema and erythema. However, these clear rapidly and the only treatments indicated are mild analgesics and cold compresses.

Second degree burns of the eyelids generally heal with no permanent scarring (Fig. 12). The main concern in treating a second degree burn is the prevention of secondary infection, which would cause third degree damage. Proper debridement of the wound edges and topical and systemic antibiotics are indicated.

Third degree burns of the eyelids present major problems. The eyelids are anchored horizontally by the palpebral tendons. However, nothing counteracts vertical contracture forces. Thus, scar tissue contraction following third degree burns frequently causes ectropion with chronic exposure, corneal drying and

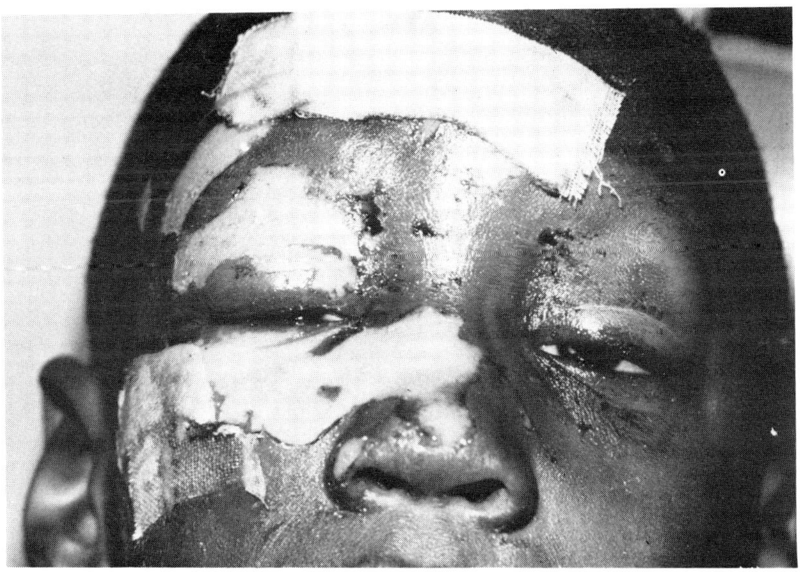

FIG. 12. Second degree thermal burns of eyelids and nose. No globe involvement.

secondary corneal ulcers. Third degree burns frequently require skin grafts and tarsorrhaphies.

Corneal and conjunctival burns are treated with prophylactic antibiotics and cycloplegics. While topical corticosteroids may reduce scarring, their use may delay wound healing and cause secondary infection. They should not be used without ophthalmology consultation.

Chemical Burns

Chemical burns to the eyelids and globes are considered acute ocular emergencies and require *immediate* treatment.

Caustic alkalis, whether industrial or household, frequently cause severe ocular complications with significant loss of visual acuity. Generally, strong alkalis are not buffered or neutralized by tears and conjunctival secretions, thus they penetrate deeply into the cornea and sclera where they cause long-term severe complications. Alkali-injured globes may clinically appear as "Greek statue eyes" or "porcelain eyes" due to rapid obliteration of conjunctival blood vessels and pearly opacification of the cornea (Fig. 13).

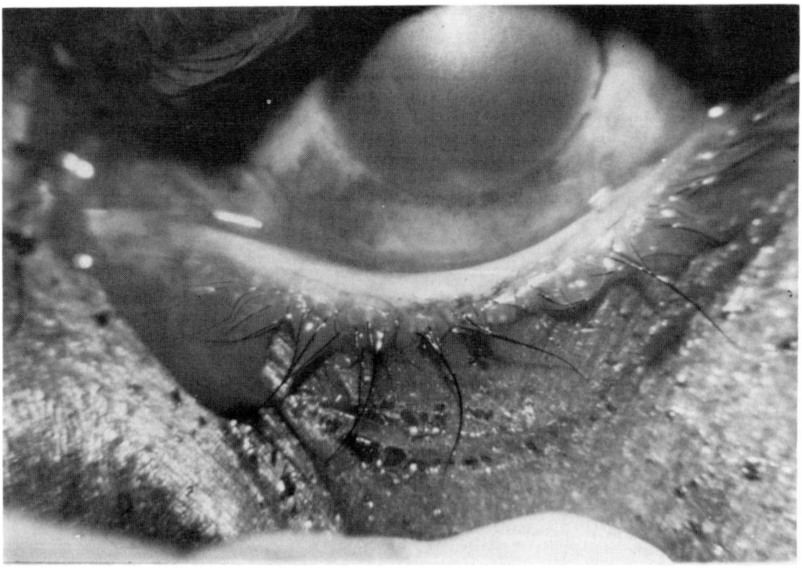

FIG. 13. "Porcelain" globe with pearly cornea after intentional alkali injury.

The immediate treatment of an alkali-injured globe is copious irrigation with whatever nontoxic fluid is available. In the emergency room, foreign bodies should be immediately removed with cotton-tipped applicators and multiliter irrigation begun with normal saline or Ringer's lactate. Often, the globe is so severely injured, no topical anesthesia is required. Other eyes may have marked blepharospasm and require topical anesthetics and lid retraction. In the home setting, vigorous irrigation with tap water or any nontoxic solution is immediately indicated, and further copious irrigation must be vigorously carried out in the emergency room. Every effort must be made to identify the chemical involved. However, litmus paper will immediately tell whether it is acid or alkali. No precious time should be wasted searching for a buffering or neutralizing solution unless it is immediately available. No strong acids should be used to neutralize the alkali since the combination may produce damaging heat. Badly injured globes require hospitalization, constant irrigation around the clock, as well as antibiotics and cycloplegics.

Alkali-injured globes may "heal" by proliferation of conjunctival tissue which frequently migrates onto the cornea and also forms symblepharon between the eyelids and conjunctiva (Fig. 14). Conjunctival scar tissue contracts like other scar tissue and causes entropion of the eyelids with resultant chronic irritation. Unfortunately, the vascularized conjunctival scar on the cornea greatly reduces the chance of a successful corneal transplant.

In other cases where there is no regeneration of conjunctival blood vessels and scar tissue, the anterior segment of the globe remains ischemic. Collagenese is liberated by regenerating epithelial cells and causes "melting" of corneal and scleral collagen stroma with resultant thinning and perforation of the globe (Fig. 15). Secondary corneal ulcers, iritis, glaucoma and scarring are prominent features of alkali injuries, and the long-term ocular complications are frequently severe.

Acid burns generally are not as severe as alkali burns. Most acid burns are caused by dilute sulphuric acid from automobile batteries. Leaking batteries are surrounded by a cloud of hydrogen ions. A spark from a jumper cable or lighted match may cause an explosion with resultant facial, eyelid, conjunc-

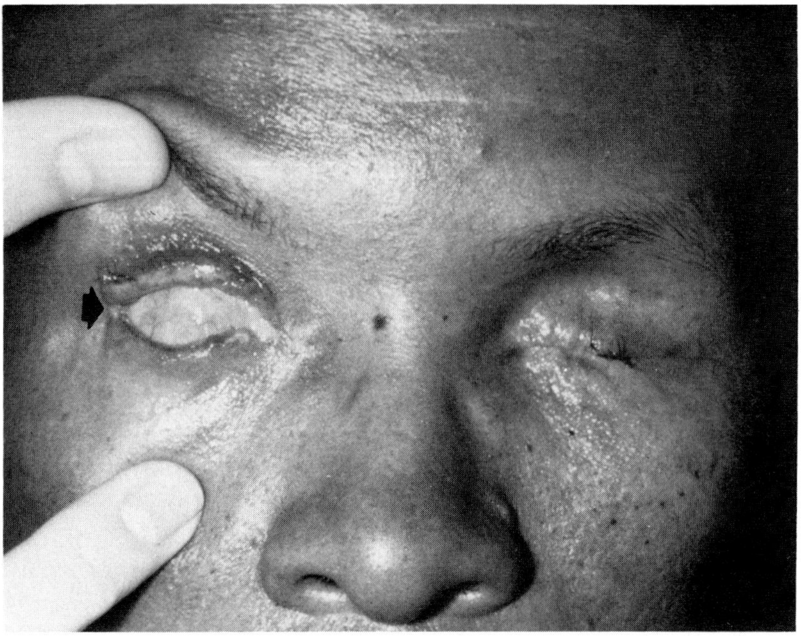

FIG. 14. Fibrovascular conjunctival scar covering right cornea (*arrow*). Left eyelids cannot be opened secondary to symblepharon and scar tissue contraction. Followed intentional alkali injury.

tival and corneal foreign bodies as well as an acid burn. In most cases, tears quickly neutralize the acid. By the time the patient is seen in the emergency room, most of the damage from the acid has already occurred. Particulate foreign bodies should be removed with cotton-tipped applicators and the surface of the eye should be irrigated with saline. However, acid burns generally do not require the multiliter irrigation required following alkali burns.

Acid burns cause a superficial keratitis and conjunctivitis that seldom heal with the deep scarring or loss of vision seen so often with alkali injuries. Follow-up treatment of an acid injury consists of treatment with broad-spectrum antibiotics and cycloplegics if iritis is present.

Mace and tear gas injuries generally do not cause loss of vision and are treated with saline irrigation and removal of foreign bodies. Mace injuries should not have ointments applied

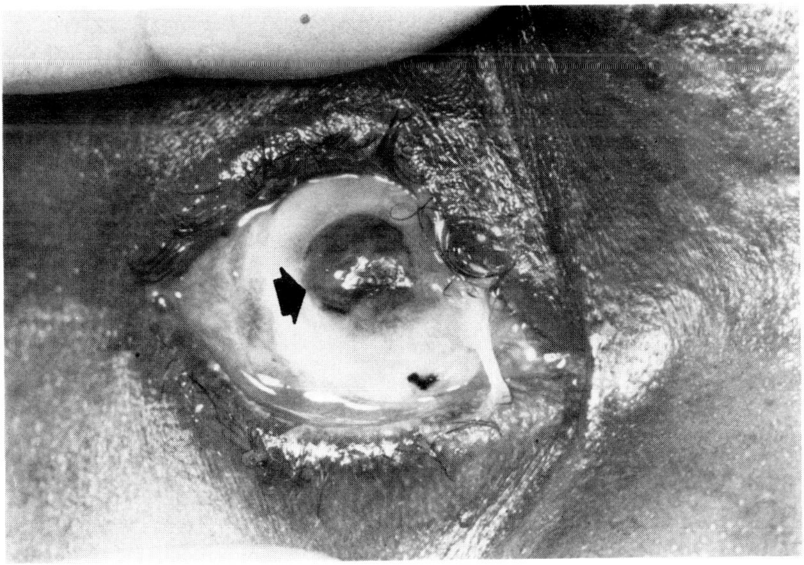

FIG. 15. Alkali injury induced "melting" of corneal tissue with secondary cataract (about to prolapse through defect in cornea).

before irrigation, because this may bind mace to the surface of the eye and cause more ocular damage.

Radiant Energy Burns

The most common radiant energy burn is caused by ultraviolet rays from welders arcs and sunlamps. Ultraviolet rays are absorbed by epithelial cells of the eyelids, conjunctiva and cornea. Lack of protective goggles during prolonged ultraviolet exposure causes a first degree burn of the eyelids manifest by erythema and edema. Corneal epithelial cells are temporarily destroyed, causing an extensive superficial keratitis. Corneal involvement may be so painful that topical anesthetics are required in order to relieve blepharospasm before the globe can be examined. Usually, there is a time lag of several hours between exposure to the ultraviolet rays and the onset of symptoms. Many patients awaken in the middle of the night with excruciating pain and initially do not relate this to an earlier exposure to ultraviolet rays.

The treatment of this common eyelid and globe injury consists of analgesia, instillation of either an antibiotic ointment or bland lubricating ointment and a firm double patch dressing to "splint" the eyelids. No topical anesthetic should be prescribed since this will retard epithelial regeneration. Despite significant epithelial keratitis, iritis rarely occurs. In almost all cases, the epithelium quickly regenerates within 24 to 36 hours without complications.

Conclusion

Hopefully, this review of ocular trauma will present the practitioner or emergency personnel with an understanding of the clinical signs and basic emergency treatment of acute ocular injuries. By no means is it a complete review of the subject and the practitioner is referred to "Management of Ocular Injuries" by Paton and Goldberg, W. B. Saunders Company, 1976, for a most complete and in-depth review of each topic.

Acknowledgments

Figures 1 and 3 are reprinted with permission from Paton, D. and Goldberg, M.: *Management of Ocular Injuries.* Philadelphia:W. B. Saunders Company, 1976.

Figures 2, 8, 12, 13 and 15 are reprinted from Hale, L.M.: Emergency eye care. In *American Family Physician.* Kansas City:American Academy of Family Physicians, September 1972.

Figures 4, 7, 10 and 11 are reprinted with permission from Soll, D.B.: In *A Guide to Emergency Care of Eye Injuries.* Chicago:American College of Surgeons, 1977.

Self-Evaluation Quiz

1. Which one of the following medications is absolutely contraindicated in any eye with a corneal abrasion or foreign body?
   a) Long-acting cycloplegic, such as atropine
   b) Broad-spectrum antibiotic ointments
   c) Broad-spectrum antibiotic corticosteroid combination
2. A subdural hematoma should be suspected following head trauma if the patient has:

a) Subconjunctival hemorrhage
b) Anterior chamber hemorrhage
c) Vitreous and retinal hemorrhage
d) Miotic pupil

3. Eyelid ecchymosis, subconjunctival hemorrhage, lower eyelid anesthesia and limitation of upward gaze is most likely due to:
   a) Trimalar fracture
   b) Ruptured globe
   c) Blow-out fracture of floor of orbit
   d) Avulsion of superior rectus muscle
4. Which of the following ocular injuries is considered the most acute ocular emergency and requires immediate treatment?
   a) Thermal burn
   b) Acid burn
   c) Penetrating ocular injury
   d) Alkali burn
5. An irritated eye with superior corneal fluorescein stain probably has:
   a) A corneal foreign body
   b) A tarsal foreign body
   c) An intraocular foreign body
   d) A bulbar conjunctival foreign body
6. Which of the following is not usually seen with a blow-out fracture of the floor of the orbit?
   a) Limitation of upward gaze
   b) Eyelid and subconjunctival hemorrhage
   c) Eyelid crepitus
   d) Lower lid hypesthesia
7. Photophobia following ocular trauma indicates:
   a) Corneal edema
   b) Macular edema
   c) Secondary glaucoma
   d) Traumatic iritis
8. An ultraviolet ray corneal burn is best treated by:
   a) Corticosteroids and patching
   b) Frequent instillation of topical anesthetics
   c) Cycloplegics to treat secondary iritis
   d) Bland ophthalmic ointment and firm patch

9. Following ocular trauma a miotic pupil usually indicates:
   a) Iridodialysis
   b) Dislocated lens
   c) Traumatic iritis
   d) Iris sphincter rupture
10. Following orbital trauma, epistaxis and eyelid crepitus are most likely associated with:
   a) Blow-out fracture of orbital floor
   b) Fracture of lateral orbital wall
   c) Fracture of medial orbital wall and ethmoid sinus
   d) Fracture of floor orbit and frontal sinus

Answers on page 289.

Design and Operation of a Transportation System: Air Evacuation as a Model

Herbert J. Proctor, M.D.

Objectives

1. To discuss the helicopter transport system and to review the reduction of morbidity for various cases.
2. To review the protocols, communication techniques and personnel training of the helicopter system.
3. To describe the equipment related to the system.
4. To assess the benefits and flaws of the system as well as proposals for improving the system.

I shall describe the air transportation system that exists in North Carolina and extrapolate from that to other types of transportation systems. We are going to talk about (1) the system, (2) medical control, (3) communications, (4) protocols, (5) training and (6) equipment.

We are parenthetically going to relate what a small group of people in North Carolina accomplished at relatively little cost. We had a rather archaic ground transportation system in 1972 and many of our ambulances did not meet the American College of Surgeons recommendations or KKK specifications. We also have a rather long state geographically, 500 miles from Murphy to Manteo. Most of our large hospitals, which have subsequently been categorized as comprehensive, are located in the center of the state. Therefore, we needed a system by which to move people rapidly into these large hospitals to receive care. Since North Carolina is the birthplace of aviation (the Wright

Herbert J. Proctor, M.D., Professor of Surgery and Head of Trauma Section, University of North Carolina, Chapel Hill; Professional and Paraprofessional Training Committee, American Trauma Society.

Brothers made the first flight at Kitty Hawk) it was not very surprising that we turned to aviation.

The System

We were very fortunate in 1972 when the Military Assistance to Safety and Traffic (MAST) helicopter program came to North Carolina. The 57th Medical Detachment of the U.S. Army is based at Fort Bragg, North Carolina. The original concept of the MAST program was that they could fly a 115-mile radius around their base. Our idea was that the helicopters should be in the center of the circle and that we would have five large receiving hospitals out in the periphery: Charlotte Memorial Hospital, North Carolina Baptist Hospital, Duke University Hospital, University of North Carolina Memorial Hospital and New Hanover Memorial Hospital. We envisioned the helicopter proceeding into a quadrant, making the pick-up and then going out to the periphery to off-load the patient.

A standard Huey helicopter was used. This helicopter can carry three litter patients and two ambulatory patients simultaneously. By 1976 auxiliary fuel tanks were installed, extending our flying radius to 300 miles.

The whole system works by telephone. For example, a physician in Kinston phones a number which has been provided to him. The telephone rings at the Memorial Hospital switchboard, but the operator answers "Helicopter Control." We have a physician on call 24 hours a day by a paging system. He answers the phone, the medical aspects of the case are discussed and assuming that it is agreed upon that it is a valid request for a helicopter, the mission is called into Ft. Bragg via a hot-line communications system between our switchboard and their operations office. The helicopter is dispatched, assuming the aviation aspects are suitable. The whole process takes about 10 to 15 minutes from the time the referring physician picks up the phone until the time the helicopter leaves.

Medical Control

Even before it became fashionable, we had an element of medical control. It is a physician-to-physician referral. The physician must first contact the receiving hospital and have the patient accepted. In 1972, we did not have any preparation protocol, but we do now. This information is disseminated to the physician as part of the operations plan. It tells about various kinds of injuries and conditions, how to prepare the patient, how to insert chest tubes, IVs, splints and how to establish airways. This is what medical control means. It also means that you always carry a "beeper" with you although it can be rather awkward at times.

Now the U.S. Marine Corps is involved in the system. They are based at Camp Lejeune, North Carolina. They fly about 100 patients a year. Although not officially part of MAST we have been able to coordinate with them over the years. They now fly patients mainly from the eastern part of the state.

We looked at 100 of our very first missions. We found that 6 of the 116 requests were refused by the MAST physician coordinator. We had an opportunity to tailor the transportation to the patient. If we did not think it was appropriate, we did not go. Interestingly, the physicians accepted this very gracefully. Two of our patients died before take-off. We had only four cancellations due to bad weather. About 96% of the time, you can fly IFR in North Carolina. One mission involved moving some frozen blood, so we were left with 103 missions in which we moved 110 patients in the first six months of our program.

Then we got a follow-up on these patients by going to the referring hospital and reviewing the charts, looking at the medic's log on board, going to the receiving hospital, examining the chart and ascertaining what subsequently happened to our patients. We had time and distance follow-up of 91% of patients and medical follow-up of 85%.

We needed to establish criteria for whether we were affecting morbidity. We used three: (1) a rapidly deteriorating patient who would not live long enough to be moved by ground, (2) was there something we could do on the helicopter that could not be done in the ground ambulance and (3) were the ground vehicles inadequate — in other words, we had too many patients, or the roads were icy because of bad weather, or we had too much cumbersome traction or ventilator equipment that we could move via helicopter, but which we could not fit into the conventional van ambulance.

Despite the fact that we refused six mission requests, after reviewing the charts retrospectively, there was a 6% incidence of what we thought was inappropriate utilization. I think that this is a very respectable inappropriate utilization rate.

The other interesting point is that 83% of the time the referring physician had made the correct diagnosis, at least the major substance of it. Having done that, it was very upsetting to note that he prepared the patient adequately only 55% of the time. Only 68% of the time did they select the closest comprehensive hospital, and 32% of the time we would overfly a perfectly appropriate hospital to carry the patient a number of extra miles to bring him to Duke University, the University of North Carolina or elsewhere.

Looking at morbidity reduction, our cardiovascular group was really a shining example: 71% of the time we felt that the helicopter had reduced morbidity, primarily because of time saved. These patients had arrhythmias, IV Xylocaine drips, they had monitors on board and things of that nature which were very difficult to do with an 81-hour EMT in the back of an ambulance. Also, we were only doing it for 35 minutes, whereas the ground EMT would have to do it for hours.

Trauma, however, was less obvious. We had about a 29% reduction of morbidity, but 40% of the time we could not tell whether morbidity had or had not been reduced.

We did not have many newborns in those days. They now constitute about 60% of our missions with about a 30% reduction in morbidity.

Overall, there is a 27% mortality in patients we fly. That does not mean we have a bad system, but rather that we are really selecting a very ill group of people. On the average we had a 38% reduction in morbidity.

Out of that initial study we made the following recommendations: (1) we want a faster response, (2) we need better hospital selection on the part of the referring physician, (3) we need better preparation of the patients before we evacuate them, (4) we desperately need better monitoring, because we are flying more and more cardiac cases and (5) we obviously need better medic training.

Communications

We began to establish a communications system where we could talk to the medics. We put 155.280, 155.340 on the helicopters, enabling the medic to talk to ground ambulances and hospitals. We also have 17 standard aviation radios installed in the hospitals that are major users. We communicate on 123.05. We have about a 70- to 80-mile radius over which we can talk to the helicopters.

This still leaves the mountain area and the Outer Banks area of the state uncovered. The next element of the system that was added was a helicopter in Manteo. This is owned and operated by the Dare County Sheriff. It is also a Huey, except that it is B model, and not as large as the one the U.S. Army flies. The Dare County helicopter flies in an 85-mile radius around Manteo and performs interhospital transfers in the eastern part of the state. Dr. Walter Porries, who is at the East Carolina School of Medicine in Greenville and my counterpart for the East Carolina program, does the medical control. He has a hotline into the Manteo office and the helicopter is dispatched. We communicate by phone and coordinate missions where I am going into his area to make a pick-up or he is coming into my area to make a pick-up.

We also became involved on an interstate basis. Most of the head injuries from the northeastern part of North Carolina are sent to Norfolk General Hospital, and there is a burn center in Charleston. The burn injury patients from the southern part of the state we send to Charleston, South Carolina. The plans are now that we will eventually get a helicopter program in the Asheville area at Mission Memorial Hospital.

The last element we are possibly placing in the system is a fixed wing aircraft, based in Chapel Hill. The transport teams will come from the University of North Carolina Memorial Hospital. These teams will be on call through the hospital switchboard. We will have a 30-minute lift-off time and a pilot on call 24 hours a day. That is easy for us to do at the University of North Carolina because we already have five airplanes. We have a pilot and maintenance pool already functioning at the local airport, which is located about one-half mile from the hospital. We will then be able to pick up newborns, high-risk mothers and selected trauma patients. This plane will not be operated solely by the University of North Carolina, although UNC is the lead contracting agent for the grant. The plane will be operated in conjunction with Duke University, Bowman Gray School of Medicine, Mission Memorial Hospital, Charlotte Memorial Hospital and New Hanover Memorial Hospital. It looks as though we will have 400 to 500 patients annually that come from more than 70 miles away from our respective institutions. This is a perfectly acceptable caseload to keep the airplane busy.

Protocols

Now that we have medical control on-line and are able to talk to the medics over much of the area that they fly, we have written transfer protocols. We are developing the concept that when the crew goes in, if they do not like the way the patient is prepared, they can refuse to transport him. It is not right to ask a medic to accept a patient onboard that he knows is not stabilized. We do not get into an altercation with the local physician. The medic is instructed to say that he has a medical control physician who authorized the mission and he is not allowed to take the patient with, for example, a cervical spine fracture unless the neck is stabilized. The medic refers the physician to the medical control officer.

Training

We are not interested in telemetry at the present time. First, we do not know if we are looking at an EKG or at the rotor blades of a helicopter. Second, the Army medics come to North Carolina Memorial Hospital for two weeks each month, spend two weeks in coronary care looking at EKGs, make the rounds with the intravenous team in the morning, start IVs, draw bloods, go to the newborn unit, work in respiratory therapy and learn about running isolettes and ventilators. We are on the verge of having a medic who knows enough about looking at an EKG that he can radio in to me and say, "I have six PVCs per minute and they are multifocal." I have enough confidence in what he is telling me that I can tell him to push 50 mg Xylocaine and hang a Xylocaine drip. Although he gets a paper strip, which he brings in to me, at the moment that I issue the orders, I am trusting him.

We have transfer protocols. Some procedures the medics can do by themselves. Others have asterisks beside them and those items, like giving Xylocaine or drugs or levophed, can only be done either with a written order from the referring physician to cover him or if he contacts medical control.

Equipment

The North Carolina office of EMS provides five isolettes, which are scattered around the receiving hospitals, plus one at Fort Bragg. They will lift off and pick up the baby. They off-load the baby in the isolette and pick up a clean isolette which has been maintained and sterilized by the hospital and take the isolette back to Fort Bragg. We have interchangeable equipment. They will usually come to Chapel Hill to pick up the transport team and then pick up the baby, so most of the switching back and forth is with the University of North Carolina.

We have Hare splints. We have Laerdal suction, MAST suits, cardiac monitors and all the radio equipment. All of that is provided by the civilian community after being decided upon by the physicians who are involved in the system.

We have off-line medical control. Four times a year I meet with a U.S. Army flight surgeon and we review all of the missions. The medics are present at this meeting, and we critique all cases. Much more valuable than that is the review that takes place right on the spot. Every morning about three times a week my phone will ring and on the other end is the previous night medic. He may report: "The patient we saw last night was really not the way the physician described," or "We had a lot of problems, we went in there and they were not ready for us." That is the kind of ongoing, informal, off-line review and critique process that is most meaningful. I can call the local physician and say, "Last night our people came in there and reported that you did not have any splints on hand and that is not very good."

This has been an overview of an air transportation system. As I mentioned at the outset, it embodies elements necessary for any good transportation system.

Self-Evaluation Quiz

1. One of the methods of preventing transportation of unprepared patients is:
   a) For the medic to refuse the patient until stabilized by the protocol requirements
   b) For good communications with the referring physician
   c) Education of physicians in the locality of the system
   d) All of the above
2. There was a 6% inappropriate utilization rate.
   a) True
   b) False
3. Giving Xylocaine requires a written order from the referring physician or permission from medical control officer.
   a) True
   b) False
4. The helicopter system reduced trauma patient morbidity by 29%, however, 40% of the time the morbidity reduction cannot be measured.
   a) True
   b) False

Answers on page 289.

Initial Management and Transportation of the Burned Patient

Dabney R. Yarbrough, M.D.

Objectives

1. To understand the approach to the immediate care and transportation of various qualities of burns.
2. To recognize and define degrees of burns and their severity by expressing them in terms of percentage of body surface area.
3. To recognize which burn is critical and requires hospitalization from those that can be treated on an outpatient basis.
4. To realize that the major role of the ambulance EMT is to transport the patient immediately and support respiration.
5. To understand type and volume of fluid administration.
6. To understand the approach to electrical and steam injuries.

A major burn is the most severe form of trauma to which man is liable. As with other major forms of trauma, the initial care and transportation of the burn patient can make a significant contribution to his recovery. Frequently what is done in the first few minutes after the injury can be of crucial importance in the management of the burn patient. Each year in the United States, there are approximately 2 million burn accidents, resulting in 74,000 hospitalizations and approximately 9,000 deaths.

Before considering some of the specific factors that are important in the initial management of the burned patient, a

Dabney R. Yarbrough, M.D., Associate Professor of Surgery, Medical University of South Carolina, Charleston.

discussion of some basic material having to do with these factors is in order. The two most important factors in judging the severity of a burn injury are the depth and the extent of burn. It is customary to express the depth of burn in terms of first, second or third degree burns, with first degree burns being a fairly superficial form of injury involving only the upper layers of the skin. A first degree burn is of very little clinical importance. First degree burns heal spontaneously in three to four days. The pathophysiologic import of burns of this depth is minimal.

Second degree burns are a deeper form of injury, extending down to the very deepest levels of the dermis, but there are still viable remaining portions of epithelium in the depths of these wounds. Consequently, if they are treated properly the second degree burn will heal spontaneously.

The third degree burn, on the other hand, destroys the full thickness of the skin. Burns of this depth will not heal spontaneously, but will eventually require some form of skin grafting to obtain complete wound healing.

Both second and third degree burns have profound pathophysiologic effects on the patient, including damage to the capillaries and loss of plasma volume, primarily in the area of the burn.

The second important factor in judging the severity of any given burn, when the patient is initially seen, is the extent of the burn, which is ordinarily expressed in terms of the percentage of the body surface area that is involved by the burn.

The rule of nines divides the body surface area into areas of 9% or multiples thereof. The head and neck constitute approximately 9% of the total body surface area, each upper extremity constitutes 9%, the anterior trunk constitutes twice 9% or 18%, the posterior trunk constitutes 18%, each lower extremity represents 18%. The total of all of these is 99% and the remaining 1% is assigned to the perineum.

The rule of nines is a very rough guide to the percentage of body surface involved by burns, but is accurate enough for most purposes, particularly when applied to adults. It is not as accurate when applied to children. The Lund and Browder chart is used in the hospital to calculate the percentage of burn with a greater degree of accuracy. Obviously, one is not expected to remember the details of this chart. But the important point is that in the infant and child, the head and neck and the upper portions of the trunk constitute a much larger percentage of the body surface area than they do in the adult. The total head and neck in a child may be nearly 18% of the total body surface area. Consequently, when judging the percentage burn in a child, this must be given consideration.

With these two factors in mind, it becomes possible to categorize the severity of any burn injury encountered. One other rule which is helpful in judging the extent of burn is the so-called hand rule which states that the size of the patient's hand is roughly equivalent to 1% of his body surface area. This is very helpful in judging the extent of relatively small burns or scattered burns. Obviously the hand rule is only a very imprecise approximation of the extent of burn.

As previously indicated, knowing these basic factors — depth and extent of burn — makes it possible to categorize the burn in terms of prognosis. Minor burns are second degree burns of less than 15% of the body surface area and third degree burns of less than 2% of the body surface area. Patients in this category should survive their injury without any significant difficulty, barring some very unexpected complication. They should have very little functional defect remaining after their burn has healed. These burns can usually be transported to the emergency room or the physician's office and treated on an outpatient basis with a very satisfactory result. Hospitalization is rarely required. Ice treatment is a very valuable way of treating relatively small burns. I am sure you are all familiar with the technique of applying ice water to burns. However, I should caution that in larger burns, ice water treatment can be dangerous because you can induce serious hypothermia if you try to apply this to more than about 10% or 15% of the body surface area. It is extremely valuable treatment for what we categorize as minor burns. Not only does it relieve pain but there is good evidence that it can actually limit the extent of the burn, that is, the injury that occurs with the burn continues for over a 30-minute period after the initial application of the burn to the body and if you can get ice water on the burn during that period of time, you can stop this process.

Moderate burns are categorized as second degree burns of from 15% to 30% of the body surface area and third degree burns of less than 10% of the body surface area, except those third degree burns that involve the hand, face or feet. Obviously, the reasoning behind this categorization is that it is critical to obtain a good functional and cosmetic result in the treatment of burns of these areas. These patients can be treated adequately in a community hospital.

On the other hand, critical burns are second degree burns of over 30% of the body surface area, third degree burns of the hands, face or feet, or those of over 10% in extent, or burns complicated by respiratory tract injury. Treatment at the scene of the accident and during transportation can be truly critical to the survival of the patient with respiratory tract complications. As noted, burns complicated by respiratory tract injury, fractures or major soft tissue injuries as might be seen in a patient who has sustained burns resulting from an automobile accident are considered to be critical burns and should be treated in a large general hospital, preferably one with a burn unit or a burn center. Morbidity and mortality are relatively high in this group and will be particularly high if patients are not treated in a facility that has both skilled personnel and the techniques and equipment available to maximize the care of patients with these very serious injuries.

With these facts in mind, a consideration of some of the important factors in the initial management of the burned patient is more meaningful. As emphasized, the burn is a major injury and, therefore, must be approached with certain priorities of treatment in mind. Initial treatment priorities are clearly expressed by the ABCs of basic life support: Airway, Breathing and Circulation.

The thrust of this presentation will be concentrated primarily on the airway and breathing aspects of the management of the burned patient because this is where the initial care rendered can make its best contribution. The circulatory problems in the burned patient, as previously indicated, are primarily a consequence of the loss of plasma volume, resulting from the heat injury of capillaries which occurs at the time of the burn injury. Also, as will be recalled, this is not a very rapidly developing loss of plasma volume or blood volume as would be seen in a patient with a ruptured spleen or gunshot wound of the femoral artery or other injury of this nature. The loss in blood volume in a burned patient occurs relatively slowly over a period of several hours. As far as the EMT's role in early management is concerned, the circulatory problem is relatively low on the list of priorities. This matter will be discussed in more detail subsequently.

Considering specifically some of the airway and respiratory problems that one encounters in the burned patient, several factors emerge as being very important. One can predict airway or respiratory problems in the burned patient under certain conditions: Did the patient lose consciousness during the accident? Was the burn a result of a house fire or other closed space injury? If the patient has a history of having lost consciousness, then obviously the problem with smoke inhalation may be the most serious problem with which the EMT must deal initially. The patient who has lost consciousness has had the opportunity to inhale much more smoke and have a severe inhalation problem than one who did not have a prolonged exposure to the smoke. As combustion occurs, a number of toxic chemicals and gases are produced that have the effect of causing a chemical pneumonitis and resulting in severe bronchospasm, very similar to that seen in an acute asthmatic attack. The diagnostic criteria are very similar in patients with acute, severe smoke inhalation.

Was the patient burned in an enclosed space? The patient who is burned in a house fire is much more likely to have significant smoke inhalation than is the patient with flame burns sustained in an open area. Therefore, these two factors are of great importance in predicting which patients may have respiratory difficulty.

Some of the factors, previously described, that may be important in causing respiratory tract injuries in the burned patient include the thermal injury and edema of the soft tissues of the head and neck which may occasionally result in respiratory problems. Again, as in shock in the burned patient, this type of respiratory tract injury tends to develop relatively slowly and is not commonly a problem that must be dealt with on an emergency basis in the field when the patient is first seen. The soft tissue swelling that may result in occlusion of the upper airway usually develops 8 to 12 hours after the burn patient is in the hospital. The most frequent problem with which one must deal in the way of respiratory tract problems in the burned patient is the injury due to the noxious gases that are produced in a fire as a result of the combustion. This results in lower respiratory tract damage and the severe bronchospasm that one may occasionally encounter.

Finally, frequently overlooked in the management of these patients is the possibility of carbon monoxide poisoning. The inhalation of carbon monoxide results in carbon monoxide combining with hemoglobin to form an insoluble compound, carboxyhemoglobin. Hemoglobin molecules that are tied up by carbon monoxide cannot then carry oxygen. These patients may then have a severe hypoxemia.

The only effective treatment for carbon monoxide poisoning is the administration of high concentrations of oxygen. If there is any question of the patient having had an inhalational injury and possible carbon monoxide poisoning, it is advisable to administer oxygen during the time of transport as indicated. This is the only effective treatment for carbon monoxide poisoning. No harm will be done by administering oxygen and one may do a great deal of good.

Some of the diagnostic clues to the possibility of a severe inhalation injury include burns of the face and neck. These patients are much more likely to have respiratory tract injury than those whose head and neck are not involved by the burn. Carbon-stained sputum, notable respiratory distress, shortness of breath, wheezing, coughing and hoarseness are all indications of respiratory tract injury and indicate the need at the very least for the administration of oxygen. If the respiratory distress is severe, and particularly if there is any element of upper respiratory tract obstruction, then endotracheal intubation may be necessary.

Hypovolemic shock in the burned patient is of relatively slow onset. Shock develops relatively slowly over a period of several hours. It is rare that replacing the burned patient's plasma volume is of such an immediate emergency nature that it must be done in the field. If it is simple and easy to start some intravenous fluids at the scene of the injury, then that is desirable. More often than not, however, all the good IV sites are involved by burn and it may be very difficult even in the hospital to get a good IV going on these patients. It is not recommended that time be wasted trying to start IV fluids at the scene of the injury.

If the IV fluids can be started readily in the extensively burned patient, one should administer lactated Ringer's solution at a rapid rate, approximately 400 ml/hr. This is enough fluid to begin the resuscitation of even the most major burn. Generally speaking, little harm can be done with the administration of lactated Ringer's at this rate over the relatively short period of time that would be involved, but wasting time trying to get an IV started on the burned patient at the site of the injury is counterproductive.

In regard to initial care of the burn wound at the scene of the accident, it is important to remove all the burned or burning clothing together with any obvious contaminating substances.

The major initial problems in the patient with thermal burns are going to be related to airway and respiration. There are some specialized types of burns, however, that may occasionally be encountered in which other factors may be of paramount importance. Electrical injuries are increasing both in frequency and severity. Presently, about 3% of all the admissions to burn units are as a result of severe electrical burns.

One of the serious effects of electrical injury is, first, the passage of large amounts of electrical current through the brain which can paralyze temporarily, or more rarely, permanently, the respiratory center, so the patient immediately becomes apneic. With no respiratory center function the patient will not make any attempt to breathe. Second, just as you defibrillate a heart with electrical current, you can fibrillate a heart with electrical current. The passage of electrical current through the body can result in either cardiac arrest, cardiac asystole or ventricular fibrillation. Both of these may have to be treated on the scene. Fortunately, except in the most severe electrical injuries, both the respiratory paralysis and the ventricular fibrillation or cardiac asystole are temporary and usually respond very easily and very rapidly to the various techniques for resuscitation, artificial respiration, that EMTs are skilled in applying.

Early proper care of the chemical burns can do much to minimize the severity of these specialized types of burns. The vast majority of chemical burns encountered result from contact with either strong acids or strong alkalis. An example of a strong alkali is sodium hydroxide or lye. Examples of strong acids are hydrochloric acid, sulfuric acid, nitric acid and hydrofluoric acid. These substances are frequently used in industry.

A most important factor in determining the outcome of chemical burns is how they are managed in the first few minutes after the accident. It is imperative to immediately remove any saturated clothing and then irrigate the affected area copiously with water. Copious irrigation is the most important early measure in treatment of most chemical burns.

Save any neutralization of the burning chemical substance for when the patient gets to the hospital. If neutralizing agents such as baking soda or sodium bicarbonate for acid burns are applied prior to diluting the acid on the skin by irrigation, a chemical reaction is initiated. This chemical reaction may be exothermic resulting in the production of heat thus intensifying the burn. It may be harmful to apply neutralizing materials to an acid or alkali burn before dilution as much as possible by irrigation.

As for classifying a live steam burn, it is really a type of scald burn. It would fall into the category of a thermal burn, as a result of heat, and then one could further subclassify it as being a scald burn, that is, contact with a hot liquid, even though this liquid happens to be in a gaseous form as steam when the burn occurs. One of the most dangerous things about steam burn is the possibility of the patient inhaling large amounts of steam. This is one of the few ways that a true burn of the respiratory tract may be sustained. The upper airway is very efficient as a heat exchange mechanism, that is, the temperature of the air that someone has inhaled in a fire, even though the temperature of the air may be very high, by the time that air gets to the victim's larynx it has been brought down to normal body temperature. So the human has a very efficient heat exchange mechanism. Some years ago, experiments were done in animals in which a blow-torch was held in the mouth of an anesthetized animal. Temperatures were measured inside the mouth of the anesthetized animal. Temperatures were measured at various parts of the trachea. As I indicated, the temperatures just below the larynx were normal. So true burns of the respiratory tract — the trachea and so forth — are very rare. But live steam, superheated steam, can be inhaled into the lower portion of the respiratory tract and cause an actual burn of the lower respiratory tract. So these patients may have a very severe respiratory tract problem when they are initially seen.

I would like to reemphasize that wound care is not of critical importance in the field. I do not know of any substance available right now that is really useful as an on-site application, because when you get to the hospital, the physician is going to have to remove it in order to evaluate the burn. My advice regarding wound care is to remove any obvious debris. For example, if the patient's clothing caught fire and he ran outdoors and rolled in the grass to extinguish the flames, you should remove the dirt, grass and burned clothing and then wrap the patient in a sterile or clean sheet. If it is a minor burn, obviously apply a dry occlusive dressing, but do not apply any topical material because, again, the physician will have to remove it in order to evaluate the burn.

Microwave oven-type burns are much like electrical burns inasmuch as the surface may appear to be very innocent, but there may be very severe injury underlying it. I do not know of any way in which that could be adequately evaluated in the field. It is going to require hospitalization and more extensive evaluation. I have heard about accidents occurring to children who were heating jelly-filled doughnuts in a microwave oven. The jelly gets extremely hot but the outside of the doughnut does not. The child takes a big bite of the doughnut and swallows this extremely hot jelly and sustains severe burn of the esophagus. These are the only microwave oven-related burns with which I have had any experience.

Self-Evaluation Quiz

1. There are approximately 9,000 deaths from burn injuries in the United States per year.
   a) True
   b) False
2. Which of the following is true?
   a) First degree burns require skin grafting to obtain complete healing

b) There is no viable epithelium in the depths of a second degree burn
c) The third degree burn destroys the full thickness of the skin and will not heal spontaneously
d) A patient with a 25% first degree burn requires large volumes of plasma to maintain cardiac output

3. The only effective treatment for carbon monoxide poisoning is oxygen.
a) True
b) False

4. Shock is one of the complications of burn patients. The following is true:
a) Shock develops rapidly usually within the first hour
b) Rarely is rapid intravenous fluid replacement necessary in the field
c) If there are no peripheral IV sites the EMT should start a subclavian line for fluid administration
d) Ringer's lactate should be administered at approximately 400 ml/hr in extensively burned patients
e) a and c
f) b and d

5. The rule of nines is a very rough guide to the percentage of body surface burns. The following is true:
a) The total head and neck in a child is 9% of the total body surface
b) It is not accurate when applied to children
c) The anterior trunk constitutes a 9% burn
d) The lower extremity represents 18%
e) a and c
f) b and d

6. The total head and neck burn in a child is 18% of the total body surface area.
a) True
b) False

7. Minor burns are:
a) Second degree burns of less than 15% of the body surface area
b) Third degree burns of less than 2% of the body surface area
c) Usually treated on an outpatient basis
d) All of the above

8. Copious irrigation is the most important early measure in treatment of most chemical burns.
   a) True
   b) False
9. Early proper care of chemical burns can minimize the severity. Which of the following statements is true?
   a) Sodium bicarbonate should be applied immediately on the scene to acid burns
   b) Hydrochloric acid should be applied to lye burns immediately on the scene
   c) Copious irrigation with saline is the immediate treatment of choice only in wounds contaminated with debris
   d) The vast majority of chemical burns result from strong acids or alkalis
10. The most dangerous complication of inhalation of steam is a thermal burn of the lower respiratory tree.
   a) True
   b) False

Answers on page 289.

Answers to Self-Evaluation Quizzes

Page 6:	1(a); 2(c); 3(c); 4(b); 5(d).
Page 19:	1(c); 2(a); 3(a).
Page 32:	1(c); 2(d); 3(b); 4(c); 5(d); 6(b).
Page 39:	1(d); 2(b); 3(c); 4(c); 5(c); 6(e); 7(b).
Page 48:	1(b); 2(a); 3(b); 4(c); 5(c); 6(d); 7(c).
Page 54:	1(a); 2(b); 3(b); 4(a); 5(b).
Page 59:	1(b); 2(b); 3(c); 4(a); 5(b); 6(d); 7(b); 8(b); 9(c); 10(d).
Page 66:	1(a); 2(a); 3(d); 4(c); 5(c).
Page 80:	1(a); 2(b); 3(a); 4(b); 5(b).
Page 90:	1(c); 2(d); 3(a); 4(c); 5(a); 6(d); 7(a).
Page 109:	1(a); 2(a); 3(a); 4(c); 5(b); 6(a); 7(d); 8(b).
Page 117:	1(g); 2(c); 3(g); 4(c); 5(a); 6(b); 7(a).
Page 127:	1(b); 2(a); 3(b); 4(d); 5(d); 6(a); 7(a).
Page 133:	1(a); 2(b); 3(a).
Page 141:	1(a); 2(a); 3(a); 4(a); 5(b); 6(b).
Page 148:	1(a); 2(a); 3(a).
Page 153:	1(b); 2(b); 3(b); 4(b); 5(a).

Page 158: 1(a); 2(b); 3(b); 4(b).

Page 169: 1(c); 2(c); 3(a); 4(b); 5(c); 6(c); 7(a); 8(b); 9(a).

Page 198: 1(a); 2(b); 3(e); 4(c); 5(b); 6(e); 7(a).

Page 218: 1(b); 2(b); 3(b); 4(b); 5(b).

Page 226: 1(b); 2(b); 3(f); 4(b); 5(c); 6(e); 7(b); 8(a).

Page 238: 1(e); 2(d); 3(c); 4(a); 5(e); 6(e); 7(a); 8(c).

Page 266: 1(c); 2(c); 3(c); 4(d); 5(b); 6(c); 7(d); 8(d); 9(c); 10(c).

Page 276: 1(d); 2(a); 3(a); 4(a).

Page 285: 1(a); 2(c); 3(a); 4(f); 5(f); 6(a); 7(d); 8(a); 9(d); 10(a).

Subject Index

NOTES

NOTES